CNOR™ Exam Study Guide & Practice Resource

2nd Edition

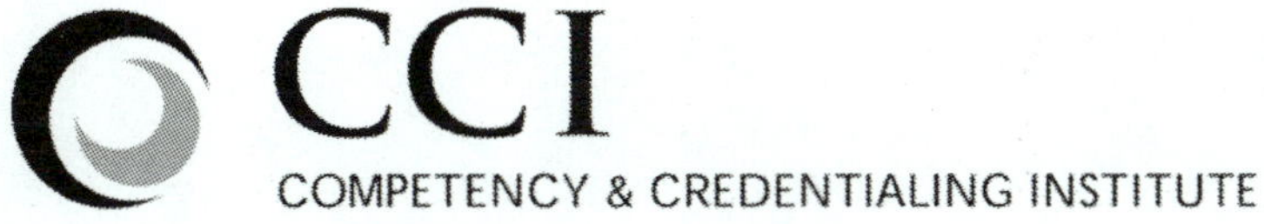

PUBLISHED BY
COMPETENCY & CREDENTIALING INSTITUTE
2170 SOUTH PARKER ROAD, SUITE 295
DENVER, CO 80231

CNOR™ Exam Study Guide & Practice Resource

2nd Edition

MANAGING EDITOR
Rose Moss, RN, MN, CNOR

PUBLISHED BY

COMPETENCY & CREDENTIALING INSTITUTE

This study guide has been developed in an effort to provide information for the perioperative nurse who is preparing for the CNOR examination. The perioperative nurse's scope of practice has been used as the overall basis for the organization of this publication and also serves as the basic framework for each chapter.

The Competency & Credentialing Institute presents this publication in the hope that it will enhance the knowledge and skill level of the perioperative nurse who strives to demonstrate professional achievement in practice.

Printed in the United States of America

ISBN 0-9755798-9-4

Table of Contents

Preface

Mary O'Neale, RN, MN, CNOR
Director of Credentialing & Education, CCI

This examination study guide and practice resource is designed to function as one of several tools that will assist you in reaching your goal of CNOR certification. The chapters in this book correlate with the Job Analysis and Test Specifications. The Job Analysis describes the overall functions and responsibilities as well as the underlying knowledge and skills that are essential to ensure proficiency as a perioperative nurse. The Test Specifications are the guidelines used for the development of the certification examination.

Chapter titles one through nine are the domains from the Job Analysis. Within each chapter are knowledge and skill statements. Knowledge statements describe an organized body of information, usually of a factual or procedural nature. When applied, a knowledge statement makes successful performance of the task statement possible. A skill statement describes the proficient manual, verbal, or mental manipulation of data, people, or things. Skills embody observable, quantifiable, and measurable performance characteristics.

At the end of the book are the Bibliography and References, as well as a list of Recommended Study Material. After identifying the areas in which you might need additional help, you may want to refer to the resources listed to assist in your preparation for the exam. The examination is constructed to reflect the professional actions taken by perioperative nurses in providing care for patients during the preoperative, intraoperative, and postoperative periods. The Practice Questions will test a candidate's ability to apply knowledge and skills to practice.

Chapter 10, "Strategies for Success: Getting Prepared and Being Test-Wise," provides information about planning a personalized study program. You will find information on the processes involved with answering multiple-choice test questions and developing skills in test-taking strategies. This chapter is meant to provide the candidate with tools on how to be successful in passing the CNOR certification examination.

You may find it helpful to form a study group and use this book as a template to plan study sessions. Statistics show that people retain more information when they read it, verbalize it, and write it, than when it is simply read.

If you have further questions about this resource guide, please contact the CCI Director of Credentialing & Education at (888) 257-2667.

Good luck as you embark on this exciting phase of your career.

Contributing Authors

Paula Bishop, RN, MSN, CNOR
Clinical Director, Surgical Services
Aultman Health Foundation
Canton, Ohio

Robin Chard, RN, PhD, CNOR
Clinical Assistant Professor
Florida International University
School of Nursing
Hollywood, Florida

Jim D'Alfonso, RN, MSN, CNOR
Associate Vice President
Scottsdale Healthcare
Scottsdale, Arizona

Cecil A. King, RN, MS, CNOR
Perioperative Advanced Practice Nurse
Sinai Hospital of Baltimore
Baltimore, Maryland

Sherron C. Kurtz, RN, MSA, MSN, CNOR, CNAA
Director, Surgical Services
WellStar Kennestone Hospital
Marietta, Georgia

Charles J. Moss, III, CRNA, MS
Director of Anesthesia Services
San Luis Valley Regional Medical Center
Alamosa, Colorado

Rose Moss, RN, MN, CNOR
Nurse Consultant
CCI
Denver, Colorado

Nancymarie Phillips, RN, BSN, MEd, CNOR
Director of Perioperative Education
Lakeland Community College
Kirtland, Ohio

Darin M. Prescott, RN-BC, BSN, CNOR, CASC
Perioperative Educator
St. Cloud Hospital
St. Cloud, Minnesota

Carol Schramm, RN, MSN, CNOR
Perioperative Clinical Nurse Specialist
John Dempsey Hospital
University of Connecticut Health Center
Farmington, Connecticut

Linda D. Waters, RN, PhD
Vice President, Consulting Services
Thomson Prometric
Lawrenceville, New Jersey

Mary Beth Zaleski, RN, CNOR
Patient Care Specialist
Staff Development Instructor
Aultman Health Foundation
Canton, Ohio

Chapter 1

Patient Assessment and Diagnosis

Nancymarie Phillips, RN, BSN, MEd, CNOR

Patient assessment is the cornerstone of perioperative patient care. The perioperative nurse views each patient as an individual with common and unique needs that can influence the surgical procedure and its expected outcome. The patient can have a set of circumstances that requires critical thinking to collect the necessary data and establish the plan of care.

Assessment is performed throughout the entire care period. The initial assessment sets the baseline and takes information from primary sources, such as the patient, family, guardians, and significant others. Secondary sources include the medical record, lab work, and other caregivers.

Learning Objectives

Individuals preparing for the CNOR exam should direct their study activities toward obtaining the knowledge and skills required to accurately assess patients and formulate appropriate nursing diagnoses. Upon completion of this chapter, the individual should be able to:

1. Describe the importance of patient assessment in the preoperative phase of patient care.
2. List several techniques for patient assessment by the circulating nurse.
3. Analyze patient assessment data.
4. Identify salient information during patient assessment that could influence the desired outcome.
5. Discuss key information from assessment data that is communicated to other surgical team members.
6. Describe three elements of patient identification that are verified during patient assessment.
7. List three primary considerations in the formulation of the nursing diagnosis.
8. Differentiate between medical and nursing diagnoses.
9. Discuss how patient assessment and nursing diagnosis provide a cogent basis for planning safe patient care in the operating room (OR).
10. Describe how patient assessment is an ongoing process throughout the perioperative care period.

Overview of Nursing Assessment and Diagnosis

The information collected during patient assessment sets the stage for the plan of care. Individual differences such as physical size or disability may require special positioning aids or mobility assistance between the transport cart and the operating bed. Age-extreme patients (i.e., very young or very old) may need family members close by for reassurance. The absence of psychological support can increase anxiety and affect coping.

Procedural activities can be affected by the findings revealed during the assessment. Conditions such as allergies or metabolic disease may require a change in intraoperative medication or irrigation solutions. The patient may have a full stomach, and the surgery may need to be delayed for several hours or the type of planned anesthetic may need to change from general to local. Chemical or alcohol ingestion could interact with the anesthetic.

A nursing diagnosis is derived from the nursing assessment data and provides the framework for nursing intervention that enables the patient to attain the desired outcomes. It signifies a standardized nursing nomenclature and consists of three parts:

- human response of the patient to health, disease, and the environment (objective signs and subjective symptoms);
- defining characteristics, such as a problem, needs, or health status consideration; and
- etiology or related factors supported by medical data.

The differences between the nursing diagnosis and the medical diagnosis are as follows.

- Medical diagnosis: Pathophysiology is determined by the physician after evaluation of medical data, laboratory data, radiologic data, and other medical processes

Task/Knowledge/Skill Statements

ASSESS HEALTH STATUS OF THE PATIENT—CONFIRM PATIENT IDENTITY, PROCEDURE, AND OPERATIVE SITE

- Health assessment techniques
- Anatomy and physiology
- Pathophysiology
- Diagnostic procedures and results
- Approved nursing diagnoses (e.g., North American Nursing Diagnosis)
- Surgical procedure
- Pharmacology and anesthetic agents
- Principles of patient safety
- Principles of patients' rights
- Preoperative patient preparation activities
- Communication theories and techniques (e.g., patient/family)
- Interviewing techniques (e.g., patient/family)
- Reporting techniques to multidisciplinary health care providers (e.g., critical lab values; medical condition; medications; allergies; implants/implantable devices; hand off; read back verbal orders; communication barriers)
- Standard and transmission-based precautions
- Surgical consent process

ASSESS HEALTH STATUS OF THE PATIENT—COLLECT, ANALYZE, PRIORITIZE PATIENT DATA (E.G., LAB VALUES; OTHER MEDICAL CONDITIONS; MEDICAL RECORD REVIEW)

- Health assessment techniques
- Anatomy and physiology
- Pathophysiology
- Diagnostic procedures and results
- Approved nursing diagnoses (e.g., North American Nursing Diagnosis)
- Surgical procedure
- Physiology responses to the surgical experience including potential complications
- Principles of positioning
- Ergonomics and body mechanics (e.g., patient/equipment)
- Instruments, supplies, and equipment relating to surgical procedure
- Interviewing techniques (e.g., patient/family)
- Reporting techniques to multidisciplinary health care providers (e.g., critical lab values; medical condition; medications; allergies; implants/implantable devices; hand off; read back verbal orders; communication barriers)

ASSESS HEALTH STATUS OF THE PATIENT—USE HEALTH ASSESSMENT TECHNIQUES TO EVALUATE PATIENT HEALTH STATUS AND TO PLAN FOR CARE (E.G., INTERVIEW; OBSERVATION)

→

performed by a physician.

- Nursing diagnosis: Evaluation of human responses to actual or potential problems or conditions by the registered nurse who is responsible for and capable of independent treatment.

The North American Nursing Diagnosis Association (NANDA) has developed an ordered taxonomy of 155 accepted nursing diagnoses that can be used to clearly identify specific responses, risk factors, and potential concerns for each patient. These can be categorized by human response patterns and functional health patterns:

- Human response patterns
  - exchanging
  - communicating
  - relating
  - valuing
  - choosing
  - moving
  - perceiving
  - knowing
  - feeling
- Functional health patterns
  - health perception/health management
  - nutritional/metabolic
  - elimination
  - activity/exercise
  - sleep/rest
  - cognitive/perceptual
  - self-perception/self-concept
  - role/relationship
  - sexuality/reproductive
  - coping/stress tolerance
  - value/belief

The perioperative nursing diagnosis begins with admission of the patient to the presurgical area. The assessment and nursing diagnosis process will be started by the admitting registered nurse. The nursing process will be continued by the perioperative nurse in the OR suite.

The immediacy of the assessment in the OR suite requires the perioperative nurse to make several nursing diagnoses concurrently. For example, the patient is lying on the transport cart/bed outside the door to the OR. The perioperative

Task/Knowledge/Skill Statements

- Health assessment techniques
- Anatomy and physiology
- Pathophysiology
- Diagnostic procedures and results
- Approved nursing diagnoses (e.g. North American Nursing diagnosis)
- Transcultural nursing theory (e.g., cultural and ethnic influences; family patterns; spiritually and related practices)
- Behavioral responses to the surgical experience
- Theories of and resources for patient/family education
- Legal responsibilities and implications for patient care
- Preoperative patient preparation activities
- Principles of positioning
- Instruments, supplies, and equipment relating to surgical procedure
- Communication theories and techniques (e.g., patient/family)
- Interviewing techniques (e.g., patient/family)
- Reporting techniques to multidisciplinary health care providers (e.g., critical lab values; medical condition; medications; allergies; implants/implantable devices; hand off; read back verbal orders; communication barriers)
- Multidisciplinary services (e.g., nutrition; wound care; social work; visiting nurse; referrals; transportation)

Formulate a nursing diagnosis

- Health assessment techniques
- Anatomy and physiology
- Pathophysiology
- Diagnostic procedures and results
- Approved nursing diagnoses (e.g., North American Nursing Diagnosis)
- Behavioral responses to the surgical experience
- Theories of and resources for patient/family education
- Surgical procedure
- Principles of patient safety
- Aseptic technique
- Principles of wound healing
- Principles of positioning
- Ergonomics and body mechanics (e.g., patient/equipment)
- Documentation of all nursing interventions
- Environmental factors (e.g., temperature; humidity; air exchange; noise)
- Communication theories and techniques (e.g., patient/family)
- Interviewing techniques (e.g., patient/family)
- Multidisciplinary services (e.g., nutrition; wound care; social work; visiting nurse; referrals; transportation)

nurse introduces him or herself and identifies the patient according to facility policy and procedure. The perioperative nurse reviews the medical record for the history and physical, appropriate consents, laboratory reports, and other medical diagnostic data. In these few moments, several initial parameters are assessed:

- Human response patterns:
  - exchanging
  - communicating
  - relating
  - perceiving
  - knowing

- Functional health patterns:
  - health perception/management
  - nutritional/metabolic
  - activity/exercise
  - cognitive/perceptual
  - coping/stress tolerance

Data from this initial assessment may identify several nursing diagnoses that may include, but are not limited to:

- knowledge deficit;
- thought processes, altered;
- impaired verbal ability; and
- ineffective coping.

Communication Techniques

Communication consists of spoken language, body gestures, and symbolic actions that convey messages between the nurse and the patient and/or family members. Each component of communication, individually or in combination, conveys meaning that provides information concerning activities involved with exchanging, perceiving, and understanding the intended message.

Spoken language is a direct form of relaying a message that should be presented by the speaker freely, without interruption. This should be a two-way exchange between the nurse and the patient. The nurse may elicit spoken language as communication from the patient by asking open-ended questions and then pausing to permit the patient enough time to answer. In the OR, the perioperative nurse has time constraints and should ask open-ended questions directed at obtaining specific information that validates steps toward patient safety, such as the correct surgical site and medication/chemical sensitivity or allergy.

Additional information is exchanged in a subliminal manner through physical behaviors, such as eye contact, hesitancy in speech, and jitteriness. This is two-way communication because the nurse displays behaviors to the patient that relay acceptance, repulsion, indifference, or genuine caring. Patients are sensitive to the nurse's body gestures because they feel helpless in the unfamiliar OR setting and usually seek security in a friendly face and a kind demeanor.

Symbolic behavior is displayed by the most vulnerable patients, often as a coping mechanism. Some patients may quietly cry or pray. Others may clutch a favorite object, such as a toy. Cultural influence may prompt ritualistic actions. The perioperative nurse should enable the patient to display symbolic behaviors without creating a judgmental atmosphere. As the patient's advocate, the perioperative nurse should represent a sense of security during times of fear and insecurity.

Establishing the Nursing Diagnosis

As the patient's identification wrist-band is checked, the perioperative nurse can use his or her senses of hearing, vision, touch, and smell to expand the assessment. The nurse can visually observe behaviors, skin condition (e.g., color, moisture, integrity), and general health. The patient's breath odors can be sensed as he or she answers questions, while the answers can be assessed for appropriateness. Nursing diagnoses will stem directly from this interaction. The *Perioperative Nursing Data Set* (PNDS) developed by the Association of periOperative Registered Nurses (AORN) can be used to establish the common descriptors for stating perioperative nursing diagnoses.

Standardized nursing diagnoses for the intraoperative period may include, but are not limited to:

- potential for injury related to transport and transfer;
- potential for injury related to electrical, chemical, radiation, falls, extraneous objects;
- potential for alterations in body temperature related to hypothermia or hyperthermia;
- potential for fluid imbalance related to overload or dehydration;
- potential for alteration in skin integrity related to immobilization, pressure, or shearing forces; and
- potential for pain related to surgical intervention.

This information from the patient's medical record, in combination with subjective and objective assessment data, can be used to formulate the perioperative nursing diagnosis. The plan of care will be built around the nursing diagnosis and should be established on an individual basis. Cultural and ethnic variances also should be considered.

Documentation of the Nursing Assessment and Nursing Diagnosis

The perioperative nurse should document and report pertinent data to the entire team. Patients may reveal significant information that could affect the surgical procedure or the type of anesthesia used. Pertinent elements of documentation include:

Date with Year and Time for Each Entry

- Complete date should be included on check-off sheets, especially multi-page forms.
- Computerized nurse's notes and OR records are generated to include the date and time of arrival to the department.
- Each set of nurse's notes and OR record should have the patient's full legal name and age or date of birth.
- Ask the patient to verify his or her identity. A family member or guardian may need to verify identification.
- Validate the correct surgical site according to facility policy. Ask the patient to describe the planned procedure and document in quotes the patient's words.
- Include medical record number and surgeon's name for clarity.

Patient Assessment

- A review of systems or head-to-toe assessment should be conducted, listing pertinent normal and abnormal findings.
  - detailed description of any abnormal data and follow-up interventions and communications
  - patient problems, needs, or health considerations outlined in nursing diagnosis
  - pathologic processes outlined in the medical diagnosis
  - subjective quotes from patient; accuracy of patient as historian
  - previous surgical procedures
  - medications or herbal preparations taken on a routine basis and last medication administration
  - allergies or sensitivities
  - known medical condition(s)
- Baseline vital signs should be noted: temperature, pulse, respirations, blood pressure, height, weight (in kilograms); diagnostic test results should be reviewed and results noted on the medical record.
- Stat phone report sheets from lab or other departments also should be clearly labeled with the patient's name, date, and time.

- The patient's attitude during nursing assessment (e.g., talkative, laughing, shouting) should be noted.
  - presence of surgeon, family, or significant others
  - patient behavior after visitor(s) leave (e.g., crying, depressed, silent)
- Contact phone number of family or significant other.
- Complaints of pain, including behaviors such as splinting or grimace, should be noted.
- Document safety measures in effect (e.g., restraints, safety belts, side rails on transport cart).
- Note time and contents of last meal.
- Document the presence of or disposition of personal property. A toy should be clearly labeled with the child's name.
- Maintain the chain of custody of any forensic evidence.

Additional Documentation Standards

- Do not use abbreviations.
- Draw a single line through errors. Do not erase.

Name and Title of Personnel Providing Care

- Include assistive personnel or transporters.
- Include other departments, such as lab, x-ray, or respiratory therapy.
- Use title designators (e.g., RN).

Summary

The perioperative nurse's assessment and formulation of nursing diagnoses are critical components of safe, efficient patient care. Each facility has a policy and procedure for the documentation of the assessment data, either on paper or in the electronic record. It is equally important to verbally report pertinent findings directly to the surgeon and the anesthesia care provider in the best interest of the patient.

Case Studies/Discussion Points

Case Study 1

NH, a 14-year-old female, is emergently admitted to the hospital with a prolonged fever (more than 4 days) and left lower quadrant pain (rated at 6 on a scale of 1 to 10). The surgeon on call plans to do an exploratory laparoscopy to rule out ovarian cyst or ectopic pregnancy, but is concerned that she also may have a sexually transmitted disease.

She is diaphoretic and flushed looking. She smells unwashed and appears poorly groomed. She admits to being sexually active for several years and to having unprotected sex with multiple partners and states her last menstrual period is unknown. She makes a comment about wanting a baby because that would make her a woman. She states that "a baby would be someone to love me." She takes no prescribed medication on a regular basis, drinks socially (admits to some excess in a joking way), and indicates she does not use street drugs.

Her affect is inappropriate for the situation (e.g., laughing, flirting, making sexual innuendos to males in the vicinity). She is unconcerned about body exposure and persists in allowing her gown to fall forward from her shoulders. Her upper arms have several healed and resolving areas of wounding and bruises.

She appears undernourished and has poor dentition. She is 5 feet, 6 inches and weighs 102 pounds. Her vital signs are: temperature - 100° F, pulse - 104 (regular rate and rhythm), respirations - 24 (full excursion with clear lung sounds), and blood pressure - 100/70.

She is a ward of the court, and her mother is an inmate at the women's correctional facility in a neighboring state, serving three years for drug possession with intent to sell. Her father is unknown. Her new court-appointed guardian is very concerned and supportive. She has been with a foster family for less than two weeks, and the guardian indicates that NH has a history of physical and sexual abuse by her mother's boyfriend. He was recently arrested and is awaiting trial.

Discussion Points for Case Study 1

- NH is a minor under guardianship of the court system. The guardian has legal jurisdiction to make decisions concerning the care of the young girl. There is no emotional bond between the girl and the new guardian.

- There are significant cues concerning NH's physiologic and psychological status.
  - Her body shows signs of abuse, which is known by the legal system.
  - She is acting out by letting everyone glimpse her injuries. She is watching for the responses of the caregivers.
  - She is acting out in a sexual manner and admits to unprotected sexual activity.
  - She is attention seeking.
  - She is undernourished and underweight.
  - She is febrile and at risk for dehydration.
  - She has an active disease process that may involve her reproductive system and affect her potential for future pregnancies.

- NH is young and has not fulfilled many facets of the

expected developmental stages for her age. She has many illusions in her mind about going beyond her current age into adulthood to avoid facing her life situation.

- NH is not practicing adequate health care routines. Her self-esteem is in question. She may be depressed.

- Her nutritional status can affect her postoperative recovery.

Describe the Nursing Assessment of NH

Set the atmosphere:

- Maintain a professional demeanor. Suggest that female perioperative nurses provide the patient's care. Patient is sexually inappropriate.

- Ask the guardian to step out of the room during the assessment process. Adolescents commonly do not speak freely or completely in the presence of parental figures. It might be wise to have another female nurse or assistant present.

- Provide privacy and demonstrate respect for NH as a person. This may give her a sense of improved self-image and may foster trust and reciprocal respect.

Process of the preoperative assessment:

- Assess her general appearance visually. Note any visual cues, such as:
  - skin coloring, texture, hydration;
  - physical activity (symmetric, reflexic motion, guarding);
  - affect (eye contact, body language, attention span, responsiveness); and
  - behavior.

- Touch her hand.
  - Note the temperature, texture, and hydration of her skin.
  - How does she respond to being touched?

- Ask pointed and open-ended questions.
  - Ask her name: note if she indicates her actual name or nick name. Adolescents commonly have a preferred name that they attach to their identity.
  - Ask if she has any allergies or sensitivities. She may not know of any specific allergies, however she may know that a substance or material caused an irritation or rash or made her sick. Her current guardian may not know enough health history to provide needed data.
  - Observe her speech patterns. Is she coherent? Does she make eye contact?
  - Observe the characteristics of her breath. Is there an odor of alcohol? Is it fetid?
  - When was her last meal? What did she eat? Has she been vomiting?
  - Ask her to describe what she is feeling, and ask her to point to the location of her pain.
  - Has she ever been hospitalized or had surgery before? Patient could have an ongoing condition or implantable device that needs to be considered in the plan of care.

- Does she understand why she is in the hospital?
  - Does she have an understanding of what the procedure is and what she will likely experience in the OR?
  - Explain to her level of understanding. Discuss the conversation with the surgeon and the anesthesia care provider for continuity of care.
  - Has the surgeon marked the surgical site? Does the marked site correspond to the documentation in the medical record and the information relayed by the patient and the guardian?

- Review data provided by the medical record, lab tests, and scans/radiographs.
  - The history and physical performed by the admitting physician should provide information about the patient's condition. The assessment of the anesthesia care provider and the circulating nurse should provide additional specific data that individualizes the plan of care.
  - Note the baseline admitting vital signs obtained at admission. Deviation from the admitting baselines may indicate a change of physiologic condition. This can be good or bad, but needs to be known nonetheless.
  - Lab work should provide appropriate information such as, but not limited to electrolytes, anemia, coagulopathy, potentially infectious process, inflammation of key structures, pregnancy, or current drug titers.
  - Scans or radiographs should provide pertinent data concerning, but not limited to organs, bones, function of vessels, perforated viscera indicated by intra-abdominal free air, tumor structures, or pregnancy.
  - Consent to treat and informed consent obtained by the surgeon should be documented according to facility policy.
  - Height and weight (in kilograms) should be on the medical record. Some drugs are administered in doses according to milligrams per kilogram. In an emergency, knowing the weight in kilograms in advance saves time.

Formulate the Appropriate Nursing Diagnoses for NH

NH is an adolescent who has several actual and potential nursing diagnoses. These nursing diagnoses include, but are not limited to, the following NANDA categories.

- Activity/Rest
  - Potential for activity intolerance related to bedrest.
  - Potential for sleep pattern disturbance related to physical discomfort.
- Circulation
  - Risk for altered tissue perfusion related to positioning for the surgical procedure.
- Ego Integrity
  - Risk for mild to moderate anxiety related to physical condition.
  - Actual body image disturbance related to lack of self-care.
  - Actual ineffective coping related to inappropriate interaction with caregivers.
  - Actual sexuality pattern dysfunction, inappropriate for age related to overt sexual display.
- Elimination
  - Risk for bladder or bowel dysfunction related to the administration of medications and the process of abdominal surgery.
- Food/Fluid
  - Actual alteration in nutrition, less than requirement related to inadequate intake.
- Hygiene
  - Actual self-care deficit related to poor grooming.
- Pain/Discomfort
  - Actual pain, acute related to disease process in left lower pelvis.
- Respiration
  - Potential for impaired gas exchange related to administration of general anesthesia.
- Social Interaction
  - Actual family coping alteration related to separation of the adolescent from her mother.
- Teaching/Learning
  - Actual alteration in growth and development related to behavior not appropriate for developmental age.
- Safety
  - Risk for body temperature alteration related to surgical intervention.
  - Risk for injury related to intraoperative positioning and tissue manipulation.

Additional Case Studies

Apply the nursing process to each of the following case studies. Extract salient nursing assessment data concerning actual and potential problems or considerations that lead to the appropriate nursing diagnoses for each of the following patients.

Case Study 2

GR is a 72-year-old male who is well known to the OR staff. He is a jovial widower who has had several revisions to his vascular access points for dialysis and an embolectomy. He is an insulin dependent diabetic who admits to cheating on his diet occasionally. His cataracts were removed last month, and intraocular lenses were inserted.

GR is being admitted for debridement of a stasis ulcer of the anterior ankle. He states that he initially injured his left ankle when he fell over his dog's leash on their daily walk. He indicates that the spot did not heal and is still open and breaking down. He is afraid he may need to have his leg amputated in the future. He is worried about his dog and who will care for her while he is in the hospital.

Points to consider in the assessment of GR and the formulation of his nursing diagnoses:
(These are examples and are not all inclusive.)

- Why is GR on dialysis? Where are his current and former vascular access points?
- What role will his need for dialysis play in his intraoperative care? When was his last dialysis session?
- What medications does GR take? How can these affect the surgical procedure? When were they taken last?
- Does he have any mobility problems?
- Can he describe why he is here and what will be done in the surgical procedure?
- What are his height, weight, and vital signs?
- Does he have allergies or sensitivities?
- How has he tolerated anesthesia in the past?
- Does he have any significant others? Are they present?

Case Study 3

EP is a 48-year-old female who is admitted to the hospital for removal of redundant skin after her massive weight loss. She had a laparoscopic gastric banding more than a year ago at the same facility. Her blood pressure is within normal limits and her elevated blood glucose has resolved. She attributes her good health to her weight loss.

Her husband is with her, and her two children attend the local high school. EP has attended several counseling sessions in preparation for the body recontouring phase of her weight loss program. She is very cooperative and eager to get into the OR.

Points to consider in the assessment of EP and the formulation of her nursing diagnoses:
(These are examples and are not all inclusive.)

- How much weight has she lost? Is she at her desired weight? Is her nutritional status appropriate for adequate surgical site healing?
- Is she mobile? Does she need help moving from the transport cart to the operating bed?
- Can she describe all of the areas that will be recontoured during the surgical procedure and by what method (e.g., dissection, liposuction, excision)?

Suggested Learning Activities

- Go to the NANDA web site (www.nanda.org) to find nursing diagnoses. Compare the approved standard nursing diagnoses with the 74 identified perioperative nursing diagnoses listed in the most recent edition of the *Perioperative Nursing Data Set.*
- Review a concise physical assessment text. Practice assessing patients by gathering as much data as possible without using adjunct tools such as a stethoscope or sphygmomanometer. What can you find out by using only your senses of vision, hearing, touch, and smell?
- Visit the web site www.nvo.com/delphipro to see a medical record in the Perioperative Nursing section with salient points concerning nursing assessment by review of systems and head-to-toe examination.

  1. Click on the Nursing Assessment link at the left of the home page under the Perioperative Nursing section.
  2. Click on the folder marked Physical Assessment for the Circulating Nurse to open the document in Microsoft Word.

Chapter 2

Identify Expected Outcomes and Develop Plan of Care

Robin Chard, RN, PhD, CNOR

Setting priorities and identifying outcomes are important functions performed by the perioperative nurse during the planning phase of the nursing process. The plan of care is derived from the nursing diagnoses and is developed through effective communication with the patient and other parties as appropriate. The plan should be patient centered and culturally based and provide for continuity of care. Care delivery preserves a patient's autonomy, dignity, and rights whereby the perioperative nurse encourages the patient to take an active role in the overall plan.

Identifying expected outcomes from the plan of care helps the perioperative nurse select appropriate nursing interventions and determine criteria for evaluating the interventions. Outcomes identify what the patient will be able to do after the nurse intervenes. Outcomes should be realistic, relative to the patient's condition, chosen according to available resources, and documented as measurable goals. Interdisciplinary collaboration is important in determining the best outcomes for the patient. Outcome indicators are the actual observable and measurable evidence used to evaluate the nursing interventions.

The Nursing Outcome Classification System (NOC) is an example of a standardized, classification of outcomes that are used to evaluate nursing interventions (Moorhead, Johnson, & Mass, 2004). The Patient Outcomes: Standards of Perioperative Care are patient responses specific to perioperative nursing interventions (AORN, 2006). The *Perioperative Nursing Data Set* (PNDS) is a standardized language that has incorporated perioperative nursing diagnoses, interventions, and outcomes (Beyea, 2002).

This chapter explains how to develop plans of care and identify the expected outcomes for the surgical patient based upon the perioperative nurse's assessment, nursing diagnoses, plan of care, interventions, and evaluation. Specific outcomes using collaboration and identifying and communicating measurable patient outcomes are discussed. Plans of care are presented according to the domains identified in the Perioperative Patient Focused Model (AORN, 2006). Three of the domains used are:

- physiologic responses,
- safety, and
- behavioral responses of the family and individual.

In addition, age-specific needs, as they relate to patient care plan development, are presented.

Learning Objectives

Individuals preparing for the CNOR exam should direct their study activities toward obtaining the knowledge and skills required to develop care plans and identify expected outcomes for the surgical patient. Upon completion of this chapter, the individual should be able to:

1. Choose plans of care based upon nursing diagnoses.

2. Identify perioperative patient outcomes from plans of care.

3. List outcome indicators specific to patient outcomes.

4. Construct patient outcome statements according to Association of periOperative Registered Nurses (AORN) guidelines.

Plan of Care

Care plan development requires multiple critical thinking skills on the part of the perioperative nurse. These include prioritizing patient problems, working within a multidisciplinary environment, developing criteria for evaluation, and utilizing evidence-based practice. Patient problems that are addressed through nursing interventions are stated as nursing diagnoses. Nursing diagnoses are derived from the assessment data and prioritized based on patient need. The nursing diagnoses facilitate the plan of care, determine outcomes, and are documented using terminology developed by the North American Nursing Diagnosis Association (NANDA). Nursing diagnoses identify responses to health problems and life processes and are the basis for nursing interventions (Ignatavicius & Workman, 2006).

The perioperative nurse is accountable for interventions that are nurse initiated while interdisciplinary management

Task/Knowledge/Skill Statements

DEVELOP PLAN OF CARE: IDENTIFY PHYSIOLOGICAL RESPONSES (E.G., INFECTION; TISSUE PERFUSION; NORMAL/THERMIC)

- Health assessment techniques
- Anatomy and physiology
- Pathophysiology
- Diagnostic procedures and results
- Approve nursing diagnoses (e.g., North American Nursing Diagnosis)
- Behavioral responses to the surgical experience
- Surgical procedure
- Aseptic technique
- Principles of wound healing
- Physiology responses to the surgical experience including potential complications
- Documentation of all nursing interventions
- Environmental factors (e.g., temperature; humidity; air exchange; noise)
- Principles of sterilization, disinfection
- Microbiology and infection control

DEVELOP PLAN OF CARE: IDENTIFY PERIOPERATIVE SAFETY (E.G., CHEMICAL; RADIATION; LASER INJURY)

- Surgical procedure
- Pain management
- Principles of patient safety
- Aseptic technique
- Physiology responses to the surgical experience including potential complication
- Ergonomics and body mechanics (e.g., patient/equipment)
- Principles of sterilization, disinfection
- Microbiology and infection control
- Standard and transmission-based precautions
- Cleaning, packaging, sterilizing and disinfecting methods
- Environmental cleaning (e.g., spills; room turnover; terminal cleaning)
- Disinfection procedures for equipment and instruments
- Handling and disposing of hazardous materials (e.g., chemo drugs; CJD, needles; sharps)
- Conducting and documenting chemical monitoring
- Emergency procedures (e.g., surgical; CPR; MH)
- Environmental hazards, disasters, preparedness, and response (e.g., fire; toxic fumes; natural disasters; terrorism)
- Principles of equipment inspection and maintenance
- Principles of product evaluation and cost containment
- Quality improvement principles
- Regulatory standards and voluntary guidelines (e.g., AORN *Standards, Recommended Practices and Guidelines*; OSHA; JCAHO; ANA Code of Ethics for Nurses with Explications for Perioperative Nurses; state Nurse Practice Act)
- Nursing research and evidence based practice

DEVELOP PLAN OF CARE: IDENTIFY BEHAVIORAL RESPONSES OF PATIENT AND/OR FAMILY (E.G., COMFORT; ANXIETY; OPERATIVE PROCEDURE; MEDICATION; PAIN MANAGEMENT; CULTURAL, SPIRITUAL, AND ETHICAL ISSUES)

- Health assessment techniques
- Anatomy and physiology
- Pathophysiology
- Diagnostic Procedures and results
- Approved nursing diagnoses (e.g., North American Nursing Diagnosis)
- Transcultural nursing theory (e.g., cultural and ethnic influences; family patterns; spiritually and related practices)
- Behavioral responses to the surgical experience
- Theories of and resources for patient/family education
- Pharmacology and anesthetic agents
- Pain management
- Principles of patients' rights
- Principles of wound healing
- Expected outcomes related to identified interventions
- Physiology responses to the surgical experience including potential complications
- Documentation of all nursing interventions
- Environmental factors (e.g., temperature; humidity; air exchange; noise)
- Communication theories and techniques (e.g., patient/family)
- Interviewing techniques (e.g., patient/family)
- Reporting techniques to multidisciplinary health care providers (e.g., critical lab values; medical condition; medications; allergies; implants/implantable devices; hand off; read back verbal orders; communication barriers)
- Responsibilities regarding impaired and/or disruptive behavior (e.g., patient/family; multidisciplinary health care team members)
- Nursing research and evidence based practice

DEVELOP PLAN OF CARE: IDENTIFY AGE-SPECIFIC NEEDS

- Health assessment techniques
- Anatomy and physiology

Task/Knowledge/Skill Statements

- Pathophysiology
- Diagnostic procedures and results
- Approved nursing diagnoses (e.g., North American Nursing Diagnosis)
- Transcultural nursing theory (e.g., cultural and ethnic influences; family patterns; spiritually and related practices)
- Behavioral responses to the surgical experience
- Patient rights and responsibilities
- Theories of and resources for patient/family education
- Legal responsibilities and implications for patient care
- Community and instructional resources
- Surgical procedure
- Pharmacology and anesthetic agents
- Anesthetic interventions (e.g., assist as needed)
- Pain management
- Principles of patient safety
- Principles of patients' rights
- Principles of wound healing
- Preoperative patient preparation activities
- Expected outcomes related to identified interventions
- Instruments, supplies, and equipment relating to surgical procedure
- Documentation of all nursing interventions
- Environmental factors (e.g., temperature; humidity; air exchange; noise)
- Interviewing techniques (e.g., patient/family)
- Multidisciplinary services (e.g., nutrition; wound care; social work; visiting nurse; referrals; transportation)
- Surgical consent process
- Responsibilities regarding impaired and/or disruptive behavior (e.g., patient/family; multidisciplinary health care team members)

IDENTIFY EXPECTED OUTCOMES: COLLABORATE WITH THE MULTIDISCIPLINARY HEALTH CARE PROVIDERS

- Approved nursing diagnoses (e.g., North American Nursing Diagnosis)
- Behavioral responses to the surgical experience
- Legal responsibilities and implications for patient care
- Community and instructional resources
- Pain management
- Principles of wound healing
- Expected outcomes related to identified interventions
- Physiology responses to the surgical experience including potential complications
- Documentation of all nursing interventions
- Communication theories and techniques (e.g., patient/family)
- Reporting techniques to multidisciplinary health care providers (e.g., critical lab values; medical condition; medications; allergies; implants/implantable devices; hand off; read back verbal orders; communication barriers)
- Multidisciplinary services (e.g., nutrition; wound care; social work; visiting nurse; referrals; transportation)
- Disinfection procedures for equipment and instruments
- Nursing research and evidence based practice

IDENTIFY EXPECTED OUTCOMES: IDENTIFY AND COMMUNICATE MEASURABLE PATIENT OUTCOMES

- Behavioral responses to the surgical experience
- Expected outcomes related to identified interventions
- Physiology responses to the surgical experience including potential complications
- Documentation of all nursing interventions
- Communication theories and techniques (e.g., patient/family)
- Interviewing techniques (e.g., patient/family)
- Reporting techniques to multidisciplinary health care providers (e.g., critical lab values; medical condition; medications; allergies; implants/implantable devices; hand off; read back verbal orders; communication barriers)
- Multidisciplinary services (e.g., nutrition; wound care; social work; visiting nurse; referrals; transportation)

of patient problems may be identified as clinical or collaborative problems (Lemone & Burke, 2004). The examples in Table 1 (page 12) show the links between the standardized taxonomies developed by the North American Nursing Diagnosis Association (NANDA) represented by nursing diagnoses, and the PNDS represented by nursing interventions, outcomes, and outcome indicators (Beyea, 2002). As shown in the examples, patient outcomes are measured by specific outcome indicators and provide a basis for evidence-based nursing practice. Evidence-based nursing is a process whereby clinicians use the best evidence available, clinical expertise, and patient choices for making nursing practice decisions. Practice based on research evidence indicates that the actions are clinically suitable and cost-effective and lead to positive patient outcomes (Polit, Beck, & Hungler, 2001). Clear and comprehensive documentation of nursing interventions is needed to validate nursing practice and patient outcome results.

Develop Plan of Care: Domain—Physiologic Responses

Physiologic responses to surgery are an identified domain of the PNDS and are defined as "the physical, biochemical, and functional responses to the intended therapeutic effects of an operative or other invasive procedure" (Beyea, 2002). Several nursing diagnoses may be generated from this domain. Body systems such as cardiac, respiratory, gastrointestinal, and renal are important areas to consider when designing a plan of care related to physiologic responses. Prevention of infection; maintaining normothermia; promoting fluid, electrolyte, and acid-base balance; and managing pain control are particular responses that warrant attention.

Perioperative clinical practice requires a skilled practitioner who is prepared in the science and art of nursing. Using the basic sciences of anatomy and physiology, pathophysiology, and pharmacology, the perioperative nurse directs the care of the patient undergoing a surgical or invasive procedure. Physical assessment techniques and a working knowledge of laboratory values and diagnostic procedures are essential in determining the best course of care for the patient. By identifying the patient's physiologic responses to the surgical experience, the nurse can plan ahead and anticipate the needs of the patient.

Using the nursing process in planning patient care is evidenced throughout the standards of perioperative clinical practice (AORN, 2006). The following plans of care address the physiologic responses of the patient in the domains of infection and pain management. It is important to note the need for proper documentation of all nursing interventions. The category identified as "perioperative nursing working knowledge" is the critical thinking that is required to successfully apply the nursing process. The perioperative nurse incorporates the cognitive, affective, and psychomotor domains of learning in clinical practice.

Domain: Physiologic Responses

Outcome: Patient is free from signs and symptoms of infection.

Outcome Indicators:
- Immune status
- Skin condition (surgical wound)
- Medication regimen
- Clinical documentation

Applicable Nursing Diagnoses:
- Risk for infection
- Risk for impaired skin integrity
- Delayed surgical recovery

Interventions:
- Assess patient risk factors.
- Classify surgical wound.
- Perform skin preparation.
- Monitor for signs and symptoms of infection.
- Protect against cross-contamination.
- Administer prescribed prophylactic treatments and antibiotic therapy.
- Minimize length of invasive procedure by planning care.
- Maintain continuous environmental surveillance.
- Initiate traffic control.
- Encourage deep breathing and coughing exercises.
- Administer care to wound sites and invasive device sites.
- Manage culture specimen collection.

Evaluation:
- Document patient response to interventions.
- Revise diagnosis, plan of care, and outcomes as needed.

Perioperative Nursing Working Knowledge:

Table 1

Examples of Standardized Nursing Taxonomy Statements

Nursing Diagnosis	Outcome Statement	Nursing Interventions	Outcome Indicators
1. Risk for impaired skin integrity 2. Risk for falls 3. Impaired skin integrity 4. Impaired bed mobility	Patient is free from signs and symptoms of injury related to transfer/transport.	1. Assess mobility limitations 2. Adapt plan of care to address limitations 3. Perform or direct patient transfer 4. Maintain body alignment during transfer 5. Apply safety devices	1. Skin condition is smooth, intact, and free from ecchymosis, cuts, abrasions, shear, injury, or blistering 2. Flexes or extends extremities with ease 3. Reports comfort during and after transfer/transport

- Principles of aseptic technique, sterilization, and disinfection
- Stages of wound healing
- Center for Disease Control and Prevention (CDC) guidelines for surgical site infections
- Pre-existing patient conditions and risk factors that may affect wound healing
- Skin preparations

Domain: Physiologic Responses

Outcome: Patient demonstrates and/or reports adequate pain control throughout the perioperative period.*

Outcome Indicators:
- Pain perception
- Cognition
- Affective response
- Vital signs
- Patient satisfaction

**It is important to note that objective and subjective data are used in assessing pain.*

Applicable Nursing Diagnoses:
- Acute pain
- Chronic pain
- Fear
- Anxiety

Interventions:
- Assess pain control.
- Implement pain guidelines.
- Collaborate in initiating patient-controlled analgesia.
- Implement alternative methods of pain control.
- Evaluate response to pain management interventions.

Evaluation:
- Document patient response to interventions.
- Revise diagnosis, plan of care, and outcomes as needed.

Perioperative Nursing Working Knowledge:
- Pharmacologic and non-pharmacologic methods of pain management
- Competency in operating patient-controlled analgesia devices

Develop Plan of Care: Domain—Perioperative Safety

Maintaining perioperative patient safety is paramount to perioperative nursing practice and is defined as "the absence of signs and symptoms of physical injury unrelated to the intended therapeutic effects of an operative or other invasive procedure" (Beyea, 2002). Due to the various types of equipment used in the perioperative setting, the potential for patient injury exists. Injury may occur from positioning, medication usage, and/or the hazards of chemical, electrical, laser, and radiation equipment. Injuries also may occur during the transfer and/or transport of the patient and the use of equipment, instrumentation, sponges, and sharps. The entire health care team is responsible for ensuring patient safety. Perioperative nurses should practice according to established standards and guidelines, participate in the evaluation of products and equipment used in the care of the patient, and promote quality control and cost containment measures. All of these actions contribute to safe patient care.

Often, nursing diagnoses are chosen based on patient risk factors. Although the objective and subjective signs and symptoms do not yet exist, the perioperative nurse identifies interventions that are directed toward prevention. The actions and interventions of the nurse may be categorized according to:

- identifying the actual risk factors or needs of the patient through assessment;
- implementing the nursing interventions; and
- promoting patient wellness.

Teaching and discharge considerations are addressed in promoting patient wellness. The following care plan reflects the NANDA diagnosis of "Risk for Perioperative Positioning Injury."

Domain: Perioperative Safety

Outcomes:
- Patient remains free from signs and symptoms of injury related to positioning.
- Patient is free of injury related to perioperative disorientation.
- Patient is free of untoward skin and tissue injury such as adequate capillary refill and peripheral pulses.
- Absence of skin redness or open skin areas.
- Absence of bruising.
- Sensory perception and motor function after surgery is at the same level as before surgery.

Outcome Indicators:
- Skin condition
- Cardiovascular status
- Neuromuscular status

Applicable Nursing Diagnosis:
- Risk for perioperative positioning injury

Interventions:
- Identify individual risk factors.
- Verify presence of prosthetics or corrective devices.

- Position patient to ensure protection for anatomic structures.
- Provide perioperative teaching.
- Inform patient of expected reactions.
- Promote skin and tissue integrity.

Evaluation:
- Examine patient response to interventions.
- Evaluate patient progress toward desire outcomes.
- Modify plan of care as needed.

Perioperative Nursing Working Knowledge:
- Apply principles of body mechanics.
- Assess patient throughout perioperative period.
- Coordinate patient care with health care team.
- Identify preexisting conditions that may increase risk.
- Monitor length of procedure.

Medication safety is another area of perioperative nursing practice that requires a strong knowledge base of medications used in the care of the patient. Because of the continuous influx of new medications, quick and easy access to references on medication use is necessary. The following plan of care relates to the prevention of medication administration injury.

Domain: Perioperative Safety

Outcome: The patient receives appropriate medications safely administered during the perioperative period.

Outcome Indicators:
- Clinical documentation of the name, dose, route, time, and effects of medications
- Cognitive understanding by the patient related to medications

Applicable Nursing Diagnosis:
- Risk for injury

Interventions:
- Verify allergies.
- Prescribe medications within scope of practice (e.g., registered nurse first assistant [RNFA]).
- Administer prescribed medications and solutions including antibiotic therapy and immunizing agents.
- Document according to policy and procedure.

Evaluation:
- Observe for expected response and adverse reactions to medications.

Perioperative Nursing Working Knowledge:
- Five "rights" of medication administration (i.e., right dose, route, time, drug, patient)
- Intended purpose and adverse effects of medications
- Patient condition and current medication use
- Documentation to include name, dose, route, time, and effect

Electrosurgical equipment is frequently used in the perioperative setting. Although there have been numerous advances toward developing safe equipment, electrosurgical injury remains a safety concern for the perioperative patient. The following plan is based upon the prevention of electrical injury.

Domain: Perioperative Safety

Outcome: The patient is free from signs and symptoms of electrical injury.

Outcome Indicators:
- Skin condition
- Neuromuscular status
- Cardiovascular status
- Pain perception

Applicable Nursing Diagnoses:
- Risk for impaired skin integrity
- Impaired skin integrity
- Acute pain

Interventions:
- Implement protective measures including dispersive patient electrode safety precautions and active electrode safety precautions.
- Inspect all related equipment.
- Remove metal patient jewelry.
- Review patient medical record to determine special considerations, such as a pacemaker.

Evaluation:
- Assess for signs and symptoms of electrical injury.
- Observe for redness, blistering, or burns to the skin.

Perioperative Nursing Working Knowledge:
- Apply principles of electrosurgical safety, routine maintenance, and knowledge of potential hazards.
- Correct use of electrical equipment following manufacturers' documented instructions.

Develop Plan of Care: Domain—Behavioral Responses of Patient and/or Family

As individuals, patients experience a range of physiologic and psychological responses to the surgical experience. The type of surgery, reason for surgery, available resources and support services, age of the patient, and cultural and spiritual needs are a few of the many variables that affect an individual's response to surgery. Surgery is a stressful event and the perioperative nurse's ability to actively listen to the patient will help establish a trusting relationship, which may reduce the patient's anxiety. Communicating with the patient in a nonjudgmental and nondiscriminatory manner may encourage the patient to discuss their fears and concerns. The perioperative nurse should maintain patient confidentiality within the legal and regulatory parameters.

Teaching is an essential role of the professional nurse. Assessing the patient's readiness to learn provides a beginning framework in which the nurse establishes a teaching/learning plan specific to the patient's needs. Through patient education and teaching, the perioperative nurse upholds the principle of respect for human dignity, which includes the right to self-determination, full disclosure, and informed consent (Polit, Beck, & Hungler, 2001). The perioperative nurse acts as the patient advocate and practices according to the American Nurses Association (ANA) *Code of Ethics for Nurses*, for which AORN has developed explications for perioperative nursing (AORN, 2006).

Ensuring that the patient has an understanding of the surgical procedure and its effects is part of the overall plan that addresses the domain of behavioral responses. In addition, if the patient agrees, the family should be involved in this process. Cognitive understanding by the patient includes describing the sequence of the planned procedure, asking appropriate questions, and participating in the plan of care. Affective responses include cooperating with the plan of care and demonstrating a relaxed, calm demeanor. Psychomotor skills include demonstration of intended therapies, such as leg exercises, the use of an incentive spirometer, and wound splinting. The next plan relates to patient knowledge of expected responses.

Domain: Behavioral Knowledge of Expected Responses: Family and Individual

Outcome: The patient demonstrates knowledge of the expected responses to the operative or invasive procedure.

Outcome Indicators:
- Three domains of learning to include cognitive, affective, and psychomotor
- Supportive resources such as family
- Patient satisfaction

Applicable Nursing Diagnoses:
- Deficient knowledge
- Anxiety
- Impaired home maintenance
- Ineffective coping
- Compromised family coping
- Decisional conflict
- Body image disturbance

Interventions:
- Note sensory impairments.
- Identify barriers to communication.
- Determine knowledge level.
- Assess readiness to learn.
- Identify psychosocial status.
- Assess coping mechanisms.
- Implement measures to provide psychological support.
- Elicit perceptions of surgery.
- Explain expected sequence of events.
- Screen for substance and physical abuse.
- Provide status reports to family members.

Evaluation:
- Determine psychosocial response to plan of care and response to instructions.
- Patient participates in plan of care.

Perioperative Nursing Working Knowledge:
- Therapeutic communication skills
- Teaching/learning strategies, methods, and rationales
- ANA Code of Ethics with explications by AORN

Develop Plan of Care: Identify Age-specific Needs

Caring for patients across the life span requires the perioperative nurse to be knowledgeable in applying the nursing process to address the age-specific needs of the patient. Psychosocial, spiritual, and moral development and developmental tasks are categories addressed by various theories in adult development (Lemone & Burke, 2004). Regardless of patient age, the perioperative nurse develops a care plan that is directed toward resolving patient problems.

The older adult is a patient population that has special needs. Older adults may be at risk for more complications during and after surgery. Physiologic changes in the cardiovascular, respiratory, renal/urinary, neurologic, immune, and musculoskeletal systems of the older adult require additional nursing interventions. For example, older adults experience sensory deficits, slower reaction times, and problems with adjusting to a new environment. The perioperative nurse may need to frequently orient the patient, allow additional time for teaching, and provide extra safety measures.

Older adults with musculoskeletal problems are at an increased risk for injuries, and interventions may be aimed at preventing complications of immobility and positioning. Vascular changes in the urinary/renal system may affect the older adult's ability to maintain fluid and electrolyte balance and may reduce the excretion times of anesthetics and other medications. Integumentary and immune changes may delay wound healing, and the older adult is more prone to hypotension, hypoxemia, and hypothermia due to a reduced cardiac output and decreased peripheral circulation.

The following care plan is for an older adult at increased risk for skin/tissue injury due to mechanical sources. Safety is the domain identified by the PNDS.

Domain: Safety

Outcome: The patient is free from signs and symptoms of injury caused by extraneous objects.

Outcome Indicators:
- Skin condition
- Neuromuscular and cardiovascular status

Applicable Nursing Diagnoses:
- Risk for injury
- Risk for impaired skin integrity

Interventions:
- Implement protective measures to prevent skin/tissue injury due to mechanical sources such as: positioning equipment, tourniquets, sequential compression devices, OR bed.
  - Identify patient risk for skin injury related to mechanical hazards.
  - Note general changes in skin/muscle mass associated with aging.
  - Determine nutritional status and areas at risk for injury (e.g., pressure points on elderly patient).
  - Use protective devices to reduce incidence of impaired skin integrity.

Evaluation:
- Inspect skin for any changes in skin color, texture, and turgor.
- Note any changes in blood supply or sensation.

Perioperative Nursing Working Knowledge:
- Physical assessment skills
- Body mechanics
- Age-specific needs

Expected Outcomes

Outcomes are designed to direct and evaluate patient care and are part of the overall plan of care. The perioperative nurse, in collaboration with the patient, formulates the outcomes from the nursing diagnoses. The outcomes serve as an evaluation tool to measure the progress toward resolving the problems and/or needs of the patient (Doenges, Moorhouse, & Geissler-Murr, 2004). Outcomes should be written in a concise, measurable, and realistic manner. Documentation of the plan of care, expected outcomes, and nursing interventions provides a means for evaluation.

Identify Expected Outcomes: Collaboration with the Multidisciplinary Health Care Providers

Establishing desired outcomes is the responsibility of the entire health care team and requires interdisciplinary interventions. Through an initial assessment, the perioperative nurse detects any patient problems and notifies other members of the team as early as possible. Collaborative management of the patient begins in the preoperative phase with the identification of the patient. Standard V of the AORN Standards of Professional Practice details the use of collaboration in patient care (AORN, 2006). Parties of interest include the patient, family members, health care team members, and other professionals. The goal of collaboration is to facilitate patient care toward obtaining optimal outcomes. Perioperative nurses exercise the process of collaboration by exhibiting accountability, flexibility, and solid communication skills.

Multidisciplinary services include many departments within the health care institution. The perioperative nurse is responsible for ensuring that all pertinent information provided by personnel within the various services is documented and available on the patient record. Aside from the perioperative check list, routine history and physical, and physician consultations, there may be additional patient information from nursing services, pharmacy, nutrition therapy, physical therapy, respiratory therapy, laboratory, social services, case management, and wound care therapy. All have relative importance in the outcomes of patient management. For example, the nutritional status of a patient may have an impact on wound healing, and available community services may play a role in patient recovery.

The perioperative checklist is a valuable tool for assessing the ready status of the patient and communicating any missing data or abnormal findings to ensure positive outcomes. Reporting electrolyte imbalances such as hypo- or hyperkalemia before the patient is transported to surgery prevents a potential negative outcome and allows time for correction of the problem. If a patient has questions regarding the surgical procedure or type of anesthesia, the perioperative nurse will communicate these concerns to the appropriate health care provider for explanation.

Hand-off communication is a specific type of patient information sharing that occurs between health care providers on a temporary or permanent basis. Its purpose is to increase patient safety. Details regarding the type of surgical or invasive procedure, current medications, surgical count status, and use of implants are a few examples of essential information that should be accurately and thoroughly reported during the hand-off period. Standardized methods for hand-off communication are an effective way for maintaining consistency and reliability (Moore, 2005). Communication should not be underemphasized in the coordination of patient care.

Identify Expected Outcomes: Identify and Communicate Measurable Patient Outcomes

Expected outcome statements and outcome indicators provide a means of determining whether perioperative nursing interventions affect the direction of care and achievement of patient goals. The ability to adequately measure and document the effectiveness of nursing care is important to establishing an evidence-based nursing practice. Analyzing and documenting the extent to which patient needs are managed through specific nursing interventions supports the premise that nursing care is distinct from care provided by the overall health care system. Communicating the expected outcomes becomes a powerful tool in streamlining the experience of the perioperative patient.

The following examples reflect perioperative patient outcomes, outcome definitions, and outcome indicators as developed by the PNDS in the domains of safety, physiologic responses, and behavioral responses (Beyea, 2002). Note that the indicators are observable and measurable.

1. *Domain:* Physiologic Response

   Outcome: The patient's fluid, electrolyte, and acid-base balances are consistent with or improved from baseline levels established preoperatively.

   Outcome Definition: The patient's fluid, electrolyte, and acid-base balance are within expected or therapeutic range throughout the perioperative period.

   Outcome Indicators:
   - Skin condition (general): free from new or increasing edema in dependent areas; conjunctiva, and/or mucous membranes pink; free from cyanosis or pallor
   - Vital signs: temperature, pulse, and respirations within expected ranges
   - Cardiovascular status: heart rate and blood pressure within expected ranges; peripheral pulses present and equal bilaterally; skin warm to touch; capillary refill less than 3 seconds
   - Renal status: output greater than 30 mL/hr; specific gravity 1.010 to 1.030
   - Laboratory values: arterial blood gases, serum electrolytes, and hemodynamic monitoring values within expected ranges

2. *Domain:* Safety

   Outcome: The patient is free from signs and symptoms of chemical injury.

   Outcome Definition: The patient remains free from signs or symptoms of injury related to chemical hazards. Chemicals include, but are not limited to, cleaning solutions, skin prep solutions, pharmaceuticals, methylmethacrylate, and tissue preservatives.

   Outcome Indicators:
   - Skin condition (wound): skin prepared for surgical incision is free from redness, rash, abrasion, or blistering.
   - Skin condition (general): smooth, intact, and free from ecchymosis, redness, cuts, abrasions, shear injury, hives, rash, or blistering
   - Respiratory status: free from dyspnea, wheezing, or stridor: SaO_2 within expected range
   - Cardiovascular status: heart rate and blood pressure within expected ranges; peripheral pulses present and equal bilaterally; skin warm to touch
   - Gastrointestinal status: free from nausea, vomiting, or diarrhea following exposure to chemical agents

3. *Domain: Behavioral Responses*

   Outcome: The patient demonstrates knowledge of medication management.

   Outcome Definition: The patient communicates understanding of medication management. Communication includes knowledge of medications to be used, to include dose, purpose, frequency, route, and desired and adverse effects.

   Outcome Indicators:
   - Cognition: repeats instructions correctly; asks questions based on information provided; states dose, purpose, frequency, route, adverse effects, and symptoms to report for each medication
   - Affective response: verbalizes acceptance of medication administration responsibility
   - Psychomotor skills: demonstrates how to care for surgical wound; prepares and self-administers injectable medication safely and correctly; demonstrates procedure required prior to medication administration (e.g., pulse check)
   - Supportive resources: family demonstrates willingness to be actively involved in medication management including medication acquisition

- Patient satisfaction: verbalizes satisfaction with medication teaching and information provided

Summary

Managing the care of perioperative patients requires critical thinking, independent judgment in clinical decision making, collaboration with other health care professionals, and an ethical code to guide practice. By using the nursing process, the perioperative nurse prioritizes patient problems identified by objective and subjective data. Patient centered outcomes are determined from the nursing diagnoses and are written in measurable terms. Nursing interventions are designed to achieve the established outcomes and through evaluation, the outcomes may be renegotiated and revised. The end result is to respond to the needs of the patient and provide quality care through evidence-based practice.

Suggested Learning Activities

- Review the current edition of *AORN Standards, Recommended Practices, and Guidelines*, with emphasis on Competency Statements in Perioperative Nursing; Perioperative Patient Focused Model; and Perioperative Patient Outcomes.
- Review the *Perioperative Nursing Data Set.*
- Review the ANA Code of Ethics with Explications for Perioperative Nursing.
- Review the literature about hand-off communication and age-specific needs of patients.
- Practice perioperative care plan development.
- Explore web sites dedicated to evidence-based nursing practice.

Chapter 3

Intraoperative Activities

Paula Bishop, RN, MSN, CNOR
Mary Beth Zaleski, RN, CNOR

Within the intraoperative environment, the practice of perioperative nursing requires a unique combination of active assessment, collaboration, technical skill, and critical-thinking ability that is unlike any other area of nursing. Versatility and stamina are key components in the job description of any effective perioperative registered nurse (RN). As one member of a team that focuses solely on the surgical patient, the perioperative RN is responsible for coordinating the efforts of all members of the surgical team toward the goal of an optimal patient outcome. This role of primary patient advocate is at the core of every action taken by the professional nurse during the intraoperative phase.

The perioperative nurse engages the surgical patient and family in a dialogue designed to provide and elicit necessary information, verify the accuracy of the surgical consent, offer emotional support, and formulate nursing diagnoses. From the moment of first contact, the perioperative nurse observes the surgical patient with a multi-dimensional view, recognizing the complex physiologic, emotional, and spiritual components present in every individual. The plan of care that results from this essential interaction is influenced by the nurse's education, experience, and knowledge of recommended practices. Interventions are planned and implemented using protective, pre-emptive, and reactive measures to prevent harm to the patient.

The *Perioperative Nursing Data Set* (PNDS) is a structured vocabulary designed to describe perioperative nursing diagnoses, interventions, and outcomes (Beyea, 2002). The language of the PNDS reflects the nursing process and defines four domains that represent areas of risk or concern for the surgical patient: safety, physiologic response, behavioral response, and health system. Understanding the concepts represented in these domains can be invaluable to the perioperative nurse when used as a model to organize, deliver, and evaluate intraoperative care.

The intraoperative phase begins when the patient enters the surgical suite. The simple physical presence of the perioperative nurse at the bedside during this entry into the OR demonstrates care and concern, and can greatly diminish the patient's level of apprehension. Providing an atmosphere that is supportive of patient dignity encompasses a myriad of activities, such as explaining actions, introducing team members, minimizing exposure, and limiting non-essential conversation and traffic. During this phase of the surgical experience, the patient is vulnerable to injury from multiple sources. The perioperative RN follows an individualized, evidence-based plan of care and uses intellectual reasoning to analyze patient responses and behaviors and initiate appropriate interventions. Throughout the surgical experience, the perioperative nurse anticipates, assesses, intervenes, and evaluates the patient's condition. The intraoperative phase ends when the patient is delivered to the postanesthesia care unit (PACU).

This chapter discusses multiple aspects of intraoperative safety including risk factors, potentials for injury and infection, emotional and sociocultural issues, and health system/institutional concerns. Interventional strategies, outcomes and evaluation tools and mechanisms also are addressed with regard to specific nursing diagnoses.

The perioperative practitioner of today faces an ever-expanding arsenal of new technology, including robotics, remote surgeries, novel applications of minimally invasive procedures, and "biologic" implant and graft materials. The days of every nurse being competent to scrub and circulate every case in every service are in the distant past. Today's perioperative RN is challenged to continually update an existing knowledge base through ongoing education. Hospitals can contribute to the enhancement of perioperative nursing practice by providing departmental competency assessments and educational offerings specific to OR topics. Some progressive institutions offer in-house support by providing certification review courses and promoting certification for all eligible nurses. Attaining the CNOR certification reflects the individual nurse's commitment to professional excellence and optimal patient care.

In its truest sense, patient advocacy consists of doing for the patient whatever needs to be done to provide an environment of safety (Rothrock, 2003). The essential focus of the perioperative nurse is to assist the surgical patient safely through the intraoperative experience. By using a broad range of protective actions, maintaining a diligent and focused presence, and collaborating with other surgical

(continued on page 28)

Task/Knowledge/Skill Statements

Monitor and intervene to optimize physiologic responses (e.g., infection; tissue perfusion; normal/thermic)

- Surgical procedure
- Pharmacology and anesthetic agents
- Anesthetic interventions (e.g., assist as needed0
- Pain management
- Aseptic technique
- Principles of wound healing
- Preoperative patient preparation activities
- Physiology responses to the surgical experience including potential complications
- Principles of positioning
- Ergonomics and body mechanics (e.g., patient/equipment)
- Instrument, supplies, and equipment relating to surgical procedure
- Environmental factors (e.g., temperature; humidity; air exchange; noise)
- Principles of sterilization disinfection
- Microbiology and infection control
- Standard and transmission-based precautions
- Selecting cleaning, packaging, sterilizing and disinfecting methods
- Performing environmental cleaning (e.g., spills; room turnover; terminal cleaning)
- Performing and documenting disinfection procedures for equipment and instruments
- Performing and documenting sterilization procedures
- Conducting and documenting biological monitoring
- Conducting and documenting chemical monitoring
- Emergency procedures (e.g., surgical; CPR; MH)
- Quality improvement principles
- Monitoring and documenting package integrity (e.g., tissue; skin; bone; temperature)

Monitor and intervene to provide patient safety (e.g., chemical; radiation; laser injury; positioning)

- Anatomy and physiology
- Patient rights and responsibilities
- Surgical procedure
- Pharmacology and anesthetic agents
- Anesthetic interventions (e.g., assist as needed)
- Principles of patient safety
- Principles of positioning
- Ergonomics and body mechanics (e.g., patient/equipment)
- Instruments, supplies, and equipment relating to surgical procedure
- Environmental factors (e.g., temperature; humidity; air exchange; noise)
- Environmental cleaning (e.g., spills; room turnover; terminal cleaning)
- Disinfection procedures for equipment and instruments
- Handling and disposing of hazardous materials (e.g., chemo drugs; CJD, needles; sharps)
- Performing and documenting disinfection procedures for equipment and instruments
- Handling and disposing of hazardous materials (e.g., chemo drugs; CJD)
- Conducting and documenting chemical monitoring
- Environmental hazards, disasters, preparedness, and response (e.g., fire; toxic fumes; natural disasters; terrorism)
- Principles of equipment inspection and maintenance
- Quality improvement principles
- Regulatory standards and voluntary guidelines (e.g., AORN *Standards, Recommended Practices and Guidelines*; OSHA; JCAHO; ANA Code of Ethics for Nurses with Explications for Perioperative Nurses; state Nurse Practice Act)
- Nursing research and evidence-based practice

Monitor and intervene to optimize behavioral responses of patient and family (e.g., comfort; anxiety; operative procedure; medication; pain management; cultural, spiritual, and ethical issues)

- Health assessment techniques
- Transcultural nursing theory (e.g., cultural and ethnic influences; family patterns; spiritually and related practices)
- Behavioral responses to the surgical experience
- Theories of and resources for patient/family education
- Pharmacology and anesthetic agents
- Anesthetic interventions (e.g., assist as needed)
- Pain management
- Preoperative patient preparation activities
- Communication theories and techniques (e.g., patient/family)
- Interviewing techniques (e.g., patient/family)
- Reporting techniques to multidisciplinary health care providers (e.g., critical lab values; medical condition; medications; allergies; implants/implantable devices; hand off; read back verbal orders; communication barriers)
- Multidisciplinary services (e.g., nutrition; wound care; social work; visiting nurse; referrals; transportation)
- Emergency procedures (e.g., surgical; CPR; MH)
- Quality improvement principles

→

Task/Knowledge/Skill Statements

- Regulatory standards and voluntary guidelines (e.g., AORN *Standards, Recommended Practices and Guidelines;* OSHA; JCAHO; ANA Code of Ethics for Nurses with Explications for Perioperative Nurses; state Nurse Practice Act)
- Nursing research and evidence-based practice

PREPARE THE SURGICAL SITE

- Anatomy and physiology
- Surgical procedure
- Principles of patient safety
- Aseptic technique
- Principles of patients' rights
- Principles of wound healing
- Preoperative patient preparation activities
- Documentation of all nursing interventions
- Microbiology and infection control
- Standard and transmission-based precautions
- Disinfection procedures for equipment and instruments
- Regulatory standards and voluntary guidelines (e.g., AORN *Standards, Recommended Practices and Guidelines*; OSHA; JCAHO; ANA Code of Ethics for Nurses with Explications for Perioperative Nurses; state Nurse Practice Act)
- Nursing research and evidence-based practice

SELECT PROCEDURE-SPECIFIC PROTECTIVE BARRIER MATERIALS (E.G., GOWN; DRAPES)

- Surgical procedure
- Principles of patient safety
- Aseptic technique
- Principles of wound healing
- Instruments, supplies, and equipment relating to surgical procedure
- Principles of sterilization disinfection
- Microbiology and infection control
- Standard and transmission-based precautions
- Professional and regulatory standards (e.g., AORN *Standards, Recommended Practices, and Guidelines;* Association for the Advancement of Medical Instrumentation [AAMI])
- Cleaning, packaging, sterilizing and disinfecting methods
- Selecting cleaning, packaging, sterilizing and disinfecting methods
- Environmental hazards, disasters, preparedness, and response (e.g., fire; toxic fumes; natural disasters; terrorism)
- Principles of product evaluation and cost containment
- Quality improvement principles
- Acquisition processes for equipment, supplies, and personnel
- Monitoring and documenting package integrity (e.g., tissue; skin; bone; temperature)
- Regulatory standards and voluntary guidelines (e.g., AORN *Standards, Recommended Practices and Guidelines;* OSHA; JCAHO; ANA Code of Ethics for Nurses with Explications for Perioperative Nurses; state Nurse Practice Act)
- Nursing research and evidence-based practice

MONITOR AND EVALUATE THE EFFECTS OF ANESTHETIC AGENTS

- Anatomy and physiology
- Pathophysiology
- Behavioral responses to the surgical experience
- Pharmacology and anesthetic agents
- Anesthetic interventions (e.g., assist as needed)
- Pain management
- Principles of patient safety
- Preoperative patient preparation activities
- Expected outcomes related to identified interventions
- Physiology responses to the surgical experience including potential complications
- Emergency procedures (e.g., surgical; CPR; MH)
- Regulatory standards and voluntary guidelines (e.g., AORN *Standards, Recommended Practices and Guidelines*; OSHA; JCAHO; ANA Code of Ethics for Nurses with Explications for Perioperative Nurses; state Nurse Practice Act)
- Nursing research and evidence-based practice

MONITOR AND EVALUATE THE EFFECTS OF PHARMACOLOGIC AGENTS

- Health Assessment techniques
- Anatomy and physiology
- Pathophysiology
- Behavioral responses to the surgical experience
- Pharmacology and anesthetic agents
- Anesthetic interventions (e.g., assist as needed)
- Pain management
- Principles of patient safety
- Preoperative patient preparation activities
- Expected outcomes related to identified interventions
- Physiology responses to the surgical experience including potential complications
- Reporting techniques to multidisciplinary health care providers (e.g., critical lab values; medical; medications;

→

Task/Knowledge/Skill Statements

allergies; implants/implantable devices; hand off; read back verbal orders; communication barriers)
- Emergency procedures (e.g., surgical; CPR; MH)
- Quality improvement principles
- Regulatory standards and voluntary guidelines (e.g., AORN *Standards, Recommended Practices and Guidelines*; OSHA; JCAHO; ANA Code of Ethics for Nurses with Explications for Perioperative Nurses; state Nurse Practice Act)
- Nursing research and evidence-based practice

Identify and control environmental factors (e.g., noise; temperature; traffic)

- Surgical procedure
- Anesthetic interventions (e.g., assist as needed)
- Principles of patient safety
- Principles of patients' rights
- Physiology responses to the surgical experience including potential complications
- Environmental factors (e.g., temperature; humidity; air exchange; noise)
- Professional and regulatory standards (e.g., AORN *Standards, Recommended Practices, and Guidelines;* Association for the Advancement of Medical Instrumentation [AAMI])
- Environmental cleaning (e.g., spills; room turnover; terminal cleaning)
- Performing environmental cleaning (e.g., spills; room turnover; terminal cleaning)
- Handling and disposing of hazardous materials (e.g., chemo drugs; CJD)
- Environmental hazards, disasters, preparedness, and response (e.g., fire; toxic fumes; natural disasters; terrorism)
- Monitoring and documenting package integrity (e.g., tissue; skin; bone; temperature)

Maintain a sterile field including aseptic technique

- Surgical procedure
- Aseptic technique
- Principles of wound healing
- Instruments, supplies, and equipment relating to surgical procedure
- Implants (e.g., handling; tracking; sterilization)
- Requirements of handling specimens
- Environmental factors (e.g., temperature; humidity; air exchange; noise)
- Principles of sterilization and disinfection
- Microbiology and infection control
- Cleaning, packaging, sterilizing, and disinfecting methods
- Disinfection procedures for equipment and instruments
- Documentation of sterilization, biological and chemical monitoring
- Selecting cleaning, packaging, sterilizing, and disinfecting methods
- Performing environmental cleaning (e.g., spills; room turnover; terminal cleaning)
- Performing and documenting disinfection procedures for equipment and instruments
- Performing and documenting sterilization procedures
- Conducting and documenting biological monitoring
- Conducting and documenting chemical monitoring
- Monitoring and documenting package integrity (e.g., tissue; skin; bone; temperature)

Test and use equipment according to manufacturers' recommendations

- Principles of patient safety
- Instruments, supplies, and equipment relating to surgical procedure
- Postoperative complications
- Principles of sterilization disinfection
- Professional and regulatory standards (e.g., AORN *Standards, Recommended Practices, and Guidelines;* Association for the Advancement of Medical Instrumentation [AAMI])
- Cleaning, packaging, sterilizing, and disinfecting methods
- Disinfection procedures for equipment and instruments
- Documentation of sterilization, biological and chemical monitoring
- Selecting cleaning, packaging, sterilizing and disinfecting methods
- Performing and documenting disinfection procedures for equipment and instruments
- Performing and documenting sterilization procedures
- Conducting and documenting biological monitoring
- Conducting and documenting chemical monitoring
- Emergency procedures (e.g., surgical; CPR; MH)
- Principles of equipment inspection and maintenance
- Acquisition processes for equipment, supplies, and personnel

Maintain the dignity, modesty, and privacy of the patient

- Health assessment techniques
- Approved nursing diagnoses (e.g., North American →

Task/Knowledge/Skill Statements

Nursing Diagnosis)

- Transcultural nursing theory (e.g., cultural and ethnic influences; family patterns; spiritually and related practices)
- Behavioral responses to the surgical experience
- Patient rights and responsibilities
- Surgical procedure
- Principles of patients' rights
- Preoperative patient preparation activities
- Principles of positioning
- Documentation of all nursing interventions
- Environmental factors (e.g., temperature; humidity; air exchange; noise)
- Interviewing techniques (e.g., patient/family)
- Reporting techniques to multidisciplinary health care provides (e.g., critical lab values; medical condition; medications; allergies; implants/implantable devices; hand off; read back verbal orders; communication barriers)
- Regulatory standards and voluntary guidelines (e.g., AORN *Standards, Recommended Practices and Guidelines;* OSHA; JCAHO; ANA Code of Ethics for Nurses with Explications for Perioperative Nurses; state Nurse Practice Act)

PROTECT PATIENT CONFIDENTIALITY

- Transcultural nursing theory (e.g., cultural and ethnic influences; family patterns; spiritually and related practices)
- Patient rights and responsibilities
- Legal responsibilities and implication for patient care
- Principles of patients' rights
- Environmental factors (e.g., temperature; humidity; air exchange; noise)
- Interviewing techniques (e.g., patient/family)
- Regulatory standards and voluntary guidelines (e.g., AORN *Standards, Recommended Practices and Guidelines*; OSHA; JCAHO; ANA Code of Ethics for Nurses with Explications for Perioperative Nurses; state Nurse Practice Act)
- Surgical consent process

ADVOCATE FOR AND PROTECT PATIENT RIGHTS

- Patient rights and responsibilities
- Legal responsibilities and implications for patient care
- Pain management
- Principles of patient safety
- Principles of patients' rights
- Preoperative patient preparation activities
- Expected outcomes related to identified interventions
- Environmental factors (e.g., temperature; humidity; air exchange; noise)
- Communication theories and techniques (e.g., patient/family)
- Multidisciplinary services (e.g., nutrition; wound care; social work; visiting nurse; referrals; transportation)
- Regulatory standards and voluntary guidelines (e.g., AORN *Standards, Recommended Practices and Guidelines*; OSHA; JCAHO; ANA Code of Ethics for Nurses with Explications for Perioperative Nurses; state Nurse Practice Act)
- Surgical consent process

PREPARE AND LABEL SPECIMENS

- Health assessment techniques
- Legal responsibilities and implication for patient care
- Surgical procedure
- Aseptic technique
- Implants (e.g., handling; tracking; sterilization)
- Requirements of handling specimens
- Documentation of all nursing interventions
- Reporting techniques to multidisciplinary health care providers (e.g., critical lab values; medical condition; medications; allergies; implants/implantable devices; hand off; read back verbal orders; communication barriers)
- Microbiology and infection control
- Professional and regulatory standards (e.g., AORN *Standards, Recommended Practices, and Guidelines;* Association for the Advancement of Medical Instrumentation [AAMI])
- Handling and disposing of hazardous materials (e.g. chemo drugs; CJD, needles; sharps)

LABEL SOLUTIONS, MEDICATIONS, AND MEDICATION CONTAINERS

- Legal responsibilities and implications for patient care
- Pharmacology and anesthetic agents
- Principles of patient safety
- Aseptic technique
- Expected outcomes related to identified interventions
- Physiology responses to the surgical experience including potential complications
- Documentation of all nursing interventions
- Reporting techniques to multidisciplinary health care providers (e.g., critical lab values; medical condition; medications; allergies; implants/implantable devices; hand off; read back verbal orders; communication barriers)

→

Task/Knowledge/Skill Statements

- Quality improvement principles
- Regulatory standards and voluntary guidelines (e.g., AORN *Standards, Recommended Practices and Guidelines*; OSHA; JCAHO; ANA Code of Ethics for Nurses with Explications for Perioperative Nurses; state Nurse Practice Act)

Perform counts

- Patient rights and responsibilities
- Legal responsibilities and implications for patient care
- Surgical procedure
- Principles of patient safety
- Aseptic technique
- Principles of patients' rights
- Principles of wound healing
- Preoperative patient preparation activities
- Instruments, supplies, and equipment relating to surgical procedure
- Documentation of all nursing interventions
- Postoperative complications
- Emergency procedures (e.g., surgical; CPR; MH)
- Quality improvement principles
- Regulatory standards and voluntary guidelines (e.g., AORN *Standards, Recommended Practices and Guidelines*; OSHA; JCAHO; ANA Code of Ethics for Nurses with Explications for Perioperative Nurses; state Nurse Practice Act)

Perform Universal protocol (e.g., time out)

- Diagnostic procedures and results
- Patient rights and responsibilities
- Legal responsibilities and implications for patient care
- Surgical procedure
- Principles of patient safety
- Aseptic technique
- Principles of patients' rights
- Preoperative patient preparation activities
- Expected outcomes related to identified interventions
- Instruments, supplies, and equipment relating to surgical procedure
- Implants (e.g., handling; tracking; sterilization)
- Documentation of all nursing interventions
- Reporting techniques to multidisciplinary health care providers (e.g., critical lab values; medical condition; medications; allergies; implants/implantable devices; hand off; read back verbal orders; communication barriers)
- Principles of equipment inspection and maintenance
- Quality improvement principles
- Regulatory standards and voluntary guidelines (e.g., AORN *Standards, Recommended Practices and Guidelines;* OSHA; JCAHO; ANA Code of Ethics for Nurses with Explications for Perioperative Nurses; state Nurse Practice Act)
- Surgical consent process

Document Intraoperative Activities: maintain accurate patient records

- Approved nursing diagnoses (e.g., North American Nursing Diagnosis)
- Behavioral responses to the surgical experience
- Legal responsibilities and implications for patient care
- Surgical procedure
- Pharmacology and anesthetic agents
- Anesthetic interventions (e.g., assist as needed)
- Pain management
- Expected outcomes related to identified interventions
- Physiology responses to the surgical experience including potential complications
- Principles of positioning
- Instruments, supplies, and equipment relating to surgical procedure
- Implants (e.g., handling; tracking; sterilization)
- Documentation of all nursing interventions
- Environmental factors (e.g., temperature; humidity; air exchange; noise)
- Communication theories and techniques (e.g., patient/family)
- Reporting techniques to multidisciplinary health care providers (e.g., critical lab values; medical condition; medications; allergies; implants/implantable devices; hand off; read back verbal orders; communication barriers)
- Performing and documenting sterilization procedures
- Conducting and documenting biological monitoring
- Conducting and documenting chemical monitoring
- Emergency procedures (e.g., surgical; CPR; MH)
- Quality improvement principles
- Resources for professional growth (e.g., *Perioperative Nursing Data Set* [PNDS]; computer skills)

Document Intraoperative Activities: Document all relevant facts and data elements

- Approved nursing diagnoses (e.g., North American Nursing Diagnosis)
- Behavioral responses to the surgical experience
- Legal responsibilities and implications for patient care
- Surgical procedure

Task/Knowledge/Skill Statements

- Pharmacology and anesthetic agents
- Anesthetic interventions (e.g., assist as needed)
- Pain management
- Expected outcomes related to identified interventions
- Physiology responses to the surgical experience including potential complications
- Principles of positioning
- Ergonomics and body mechanics (e.g., patient; equipment)
- Instruments, supplies, and equipment relating to surgical procedure)
- Implants (e.g., handling; tracking; sterilization)
- Documentation of all nursing interventions
- Environmental factors (e.g., temperature; humidity; air exchange; noise)
- Communication theories and techniques (e.g., patient/family)
- Reporting techniques to multidisciplinary health care providers (e.g., critical lab values; medical condition; medications; allergies; implants/implantable devices; hand off; read back verbal orders; communication barriers)
- Performing and documenting sterilization procedures
- Conducting and documenting biological monitoring
- Conducting and documenting chemical monitoring
- Emergency procedures (e.g., surgical; CPR; MH)
- Quality improvement principles
- Resources for professional growth (e.g., *Perioperative Nursing Data Set* [PNDS]; computer skills)

DOCUMENT INTRAOPERATIVE ACTIVITIES: RECORD UNUSUAL OCCURRENCES AND/OR VARIANCES IN CARE

- Legal responsibilities and implications for patient care
- Surgical procedure
- Anesthetic interventions (e.g., assist as needed)
- Principles of patient safety
- Principles of patients' rights
- Documentation of all nursing interventions
- Reporting techniques to multidisciplinary health care providers (e.g., critical lab values; medical condition; medications; allergies; implants/implantable devices; hand off; read back verbal orders; communication barriers)
- Postoperative complications
- Emergency procedures (e.g., surgical; CPR; MH)
- Environmental hazards, disasters, preparedness, and response (e.g., fire; toxic fumes; natural disasters; terrorism)
- Regulatory standards and voluntary guidelines (e.g., AORN *Standards, Recommended Practices and Guidelines;* OSHA; JCAHO; ANA Code of Ethics for Nurses with Explications for Perioperative Nurses; state Nurse Practice Act)
- Responsibilities regarding impaired and/or disruptive behavior (e.g., patient/family; multidisciplinary health care team members)

DOCUMENT INTRAOPERATIVE ACTIVITIES: DOCUMENT MAINTENANCE OF A SAFE ENVIRONMENT

- Health assessment techniques
- Approved nursing diagnoses (e.g., North American Nursing Diagnosis)
- Behavioral responses to the surgical experience
- Patient rights and responsibilities
- Legal responsibilities and implications for patient care
- Principles of patient safety
- Aseptic technique
- Principles of patients' rights
- Principles of wound healing
- Preoperative patient preparation activities
- Expected outcomes related to identified interventions
- Physiology responses to the surgical experience including potential complications
- Principles of positioning
- Ergonomics and body mechanics (e.g., patient/equipment)
- Documentation of all nursing interventions
- Environmental factors (e.g., temperature; humidity; air exchange; noise)
- Professional and regulatory standards and voluntary guidelines (e.g., AORN *Standards, Recommended Practices and Guidelines;* Association for the Advancement of Medical Instrumentation [AAMI])

DOCUMENT INTRAOPERATIVE ACTIVITIES: DOCUMENT SPECIMENS AND DISPOSITION OF THE SPECIMENS

- Diagnostic procedures and results
- Legal responsibilities and implications for patient care
- Surgical procedure
- Aseptic technique
- Principles of wound healing
- Requirements of handling specimens
- Documentation of all nursing interventions
- Multidisciplinary services (e.g., nutrition; wound care; social work; visiting nurse; referrals; transportation)
- Microbiology and infection control
- Standard and transmission-based precautions
- Emergency procedures (e.g., surgical; CPR; MH)
- Quality improvement principles

Task/Knowledge/Skill Statements

- Regulatory standards and voluntary guidelines (e.g., AORN *Standards, Recommended Practices and Guidelines;* OSHA; JCAHO; ANA Code of Ethics for Nurses with Explications for Perioperative Nurses; state Nurse Practice Act

Document Intraoperative Activities: document solutions used and medications administered

- Health assessment techniques
- Diagnostic procedures and results
- Transcultural nursing theory (e.g., cultural and ethnic influences; family patterns; spiritually and related practices)
- Patient rights and responsibilities
- Legal responsibilities and implications for patient care
- Surgical procedure
- Pharmacology and anesthetic agents
- Anesthetic interventions (e.g., assist as needed)
- Pain management
- Aseptic technique
- Principles of wound healing
- Physiology responses to the surgical experience including potential complications
- Documentation of all nursing interventions
- Reporting techniques to multidisciplinary health care providers (e.g., critical lab values; medical condition; medications; allergies; implants/implantable devices; hand off; read back verbal orders; communication barriers)
- Multidisciplinary services (e.g., nutrition; wound care; social work; visiting nurse; referrals; transportation)
- Emergency procedures (e.g., surgical; CPR; MH)
- Quality improvement principles
- Regulatory standards and voluntary guidelines (e.g., AORN *Standards, Recommended Practices and Guidelines;* OSHA; JCAHO; ANA Code of Ethics for Nurses with Explications for Perioperative Nurses; state Nurse Practice Act)
- Surgical consent process

Document Intraoperative Activities: Document patient outcomes

- Diagnostic procedures and results
- Behavioral responses to the surgical experience
- Legal responsibilities and implications for patient care
- Surgical procedure
- Pain management
- Principles of wound healing
- Expected outcomes related to identified interventions
- Physiology responses to the surgical experience including potential complication
- Principles of positioning
- Ergonomics and body mechanics (e.g., patient/equipment)
- Documentation of all nursing interventions
- Reporting techniques to multidisciplinary health care providers (e.g., critical lab values; medical condition; medications; allergies; implants/implantable devices; hand off; read back verbal orders; communication barriers)
- Postoperative complication
- Multidisciplinary services (e.g., nutrition; wound care; social work; visiting nurse; referrals; transportation)
- Conducting and documenting biological monitoring
- Quality improvement principles
- Regulatory standards and voluntary guidelines (e.g., AORN *Standards, Recommended Practices and Guidelines;* OSHA; JCAHO; ANA Code of Ethics for Nurses with Explications for Perioperative Nurses; state Nurse Practice Act)
- Resources for professional growth (e.g., *Perioperative Nursing Data Set* [PNDS]; computer skills)
- Nursing research and evidence-based practice

Document Intraoperative Activities: Document surgical wound classification

- Anatomy and physiology
- Pathophysiology
- Legal responsibilities and implications for patient care
- Surgical procedure
- Principles of patient safety
- Aseptic technique
- Principles of wound healing
- Preoperative patient preparation activities
- Expected outcomes related to identified interventions
- Physiology responses to the surgical experience including potential complications
- Implants (e.g., handling; tracking; sterilization)
- Documentation of all nursing interventions
- Environmental factors (e.g., temperature; humidity; air exchange; noise)
- Postoperative complications
- Multidisciplinary services (e.g., nutrition; wound care; social work; visiting nurse; referrals; transportation)
- Microbiology and infection control
- Standard and transmission-based precautions
- Quality improvement principles

Task/Knowledge/Skill Statements

- Regulatory standards and voluntary guidelines (e.g., AORN *Standards, Recommended Practices and Guidelines;* OSHA; JCAHO; ANA Code of Ethics for Nurses with Explications for Perioperative Nurses; state Nurse Practice Act)

Document Intraoperative Activities: Document implanted or explanted devices

- Diagnostic procedures and results
- Surgical procedure
- Principles of patient safety
- Aseptic technique
- Expected outcomes related to identified interventions
- Physiology responses to the surgical experience including potential complications
- Implants (e.g., handling; tracking; sterilization)
- Requirements of handling specimens
- Reporting techniques to multidisciplinary health care providers (e.g., critical lab values; medical condition; medications; allergies; implants/implantable devices; hand off; read back verbal orders; communication barriers)
- Microbiology and infection control
- Documentation of sterilization, biological and chemical monitoring
- Performing and documenting sterilization procedures
- Conducting and documenting biological monitoring
- Conducting and documenting chemical monitoring
- Quality improvement principles
- Regulatory standards and voluntary guidelines (e.g., AORN *Standards, Recommended Practices and Guidelines;* OSHA; JCAHO; ANA Code of Ethics for Nurses with Explications for Perioperative Nurses; state Nurse Practice Act)
- Nursing research and evidence-based practice

Document Intraoperative Activities: Document counts

- Approved nursing diagnoses (e.g., North American Nursing Diagnosis)
- Patient rights and responsibilities
- Legal responsibilities and implications for patient care
- Surgical procedure
- Principles of patient safety
- Principles of patients' rights
- Principles of wound healing
- Expected outcomes related to identified interventions
- Physiology responses to the surgical experience including potential complications
- Instruments, supplies, and equipment relating to surgical procedure
- Documentation of all nursing interventions
- Reporting techniques to multidisciplinary health care providers (e.g., critical lab values; medical condition; medications; allergies; implants/implantable devices; hand off; read back verbal orders; communication barriers)
- Quality improvement principles
- Regulatory standards and voluntary guidelines (e.g., AORN *Standards, Recommended Practices and Guidelines;* OSHA; JCAHO; ANA Code of Ethics for Nurses with Explications for Perioperative Nurses; state Nurse Practice Act)
- Resources for professional growth (e.g., *Perioperative Nursing Data Set* [PNDS]; computer skills)
- Nursing research and evidence-based practice

Document Intraoperative Activities: Document Universal protocol (e.g., time out)

- Patient rights and responsibilities
- Legal responsibilities and implications for patient care
- Surgical procedure
- Principles of patient safety
- Preoperative patient preparation activities
- Expected outcomes related to identified interventions
- Physiology responses to the surgical experience including potential complications
- Documentation of all nursing interventions
- Communication theories and techniques (e.g., patient/family)
- Reporting techniques to multidisciplinary health care providers (e.g., critical lab values; medical condition; medications; allergies; implants/implantable devices; hand off; read back verbal orders; communication barriers)
- Postoperative complications
- Quality improvement principles
- Basic management techniques and delegation
- Regulatory standards and voluntary guidelines (e.g., AORN *Standards, Recommended Practices and Guidelines;* OSHA; JCAHO; ANA Code of Ethics for Nurses with Explications for Perioperative Nurses; state Nurse Practice Act)
- Surgical consent process
- Responsibilities regarding impaired and/or disruptive behavior (e.g., patient/family; multidisciplinary health care team members)

(continued from page 19)

team members, the RN responsible for the care of the surgical patient can accomplish the primary goal of an optimal patient outcome.

Learning Objectives

Individuals preparing for the CNOR exam should focus study toward gaining the knowledge and skills necessary to perform intraoperative activities. Upon completion of this chapter, the individual should be able to:

1. Define the intraoperative phase as it relates to the perioperative nurse's role in patient responses and outcomes.

2. Identify activities required of the perioperative nurse in providing care during the intraoperative phase.

3. Discuss the physiological responses to surgery, infection, anesthetic agents, and medications.

4. Outline procedures for specimen handling, medication labeling, and equipment use as identified by regulatory agencies and standards.

5. Identify appropriate behaviors for safeguarding the patient physically and emotionally throughout the intraoperative phase.

6. Describe appropriate documentation of actions and nursing care performed during the intraoperative phase.

Overview of Intraoperative Nursing Activities

There are three phases in the surgical experience: preoperative, intraoperative, and postoperative. This chapter focuses on the intraoperative phase of surgery and the nursing activities within this phase. The intraoperative phase begins when the patient enters the OR and ends with the transfer to the PACU (Spry, 2005). During this phase, the patient receives anesthetic agents, is positioned, is prepped and draped, and undergoes the surgical procedure. The perioperative nurse focuses attention on patient safety, prevention of infection, facilitation of the surgical procedure, and promoting positive patient outcomes. The perioperative nurse functions in multiple roles during this intraoperative phase, maintaining primary focus on the patient at all times.

Monitor and Intervene to Optimize Physiologic Responses

Physiologic responses occur throughout the surgical experience and include responses to anesthesia, positioning, the surgical procedure, and the environment. The perioperative nurse is responsible for observing and applying appropriate interventions related to these responses. An awareness of some of the significant responses and interventions supports excellent perioperative patient care.

Infection

The perioperative nurse plays a very important role in the prevention of infection in surgical patients. A surgical site infection (SSI) is any infectious process that involves the surgical incision or area of surgery. Approximately 14% to 16% of hospital acquired, or nosocomial, infections are SSIs (MedQIC, 2006). SSIs can result in increased costs, extended hospital stays, and even death.

The authority on etiology, prevention, and surveillance of surgical site infections is the Centers for Disease Control and Prevention (CDC). This organization has numerous guidelines on infection control and provides a great source of information for developing infection prevention strategies in health care organizations. Two important publications from the CDC include the *Guidelines for Prevention of Surgical Site Infection* and *Guideline for Hand Hygiene in Healthcare Settings* (CDC, 2006).

Surgical infection prevention is such an important aspect of care that the Centers for Medicare and Medicaid Services (CMS) have focused much of their attention on this area. The Surgical Care Improvement Project (SCIP) is a partnership of organizations dedicated to improving outcomes in surgical patients. The goal of SCIP is to reduce surgical complication incidents by 25% by the year 2010 (MedQIC, 2006). One entire section of the SCIP protocol is dedicated to prevention of surgical site infections. Two areas of focus in SCIP include antibiotic administration and proper hair removal. The perioperative nurse should take responsibility for verifying that preoperative prophylactic antibiotics are given as ordered within the period appropriate for the particular antibiotic. The nurse also has a role in providing the proper means of hair removal, using either clippers or a depilatory. Educating staff and physicians on the quality measures also can be integrated into the perioperative nurse's activities.

Observing the basic rules of asepsis is the most important action the perioperative nurse can perform to help prevent infection. The perioperative nurse should ensure that all supplies are sterile before opening and using them. Knowledge of sterilization practices and controls is an important aspect of asepsis. Avoiding contamination of the sterile field and adhering to the old adage, "if in doubt, throw it out" are essential rules of perioperative practice. Surgical conscience is paramount in the surgical setting and a basic competency of any surgical nurse. The perioperative nurse should be aware of the surroundings and the movement of people in the surgical suite at all times, monitoring the aseptic practice of the surgical team members. Review of and adherence to the AORN Recommended Practices for Surgical Attire, Skin Preparation of Patients, and Surgical Hand Antisepsis (AORN, 2006) will help prevent infections.

Quality

Assurance of appropriate interventions is measured through quality indicators. The SCIP measures are some of those aspects of quality that are captured to ensure optimal postoperative outcomes. Reporting to the CMS on these SCIP measures provides the general public information that can be used to determine the best place to access health care. Quality measures can include any aspect of care that is of concern to the practitioner. The perioperative nurse has a valuable role in identifying opportunities for improvement and supporting and implementing changes to improve quality.

Principles of Wound Healing

A surgical patient may experience a wound either caused by trauma or intentionally created by the surgeon. In either case, the wound must be repaired and allowed to heal. Wounds heal by primary or secondary intention. A sutured surgical incision is an example of healing by primary intention: wound edges are closed and healing takes place along that suture line. A large gaping wound is an example of healing by secondary intention, in which tissue must regenerate from inside and work out to the surface.

Wounds heal in three phases: inflammatory phase, proliferative phase, and remodeling phase. The inflammatory phase begins at the time of injury and creates the environment needed for proper wound healing to take place. Hemostatic processes begin to initiate blood clotting and white blood cells migrate to the wound area. In the proliferative phase, usually two to three days after injury, the wound begins healing by primary intention; building new tissue to fill in wound space. This is the phase in which granulation tissue develops and can last as long as three weeks (Porth, 1998). The final phase is the remodeling phase. This can continue for six months to two years and involves continued remodeling of the scar tissue (Porth, 1998).

Wounds must have adequate blood flow and oxygen to heal properly. Blood flow to the area of the wound provides nutrients to the cells and removes debris, bacteria, and toxins. Oxygen nourishes the cells so that adequate collagen can form. If a wound becomes ischemic, infection is likely to develop.

The perioperative nurse supports wound healing by providing sterile supplies to close and dress the wound to avoid introducing bacteria into the wound. The nurse ensures proper positioning to avoid pressure on or near the surgical site. The anesthesia care provider supplies adequate oxygenation; however, the perioperative nurse monitors the patient's responses as well.

Monitor and Intervene to Provide Patient Safety

Patient safety is of primary importance, and the perioperative nurse is responsible for promoting safety during the intraoperative phase. The Joint Commission on the Accreditation of Healthcare Organizations (JCAHO) focuses on patient safety and updates the National Patient Safety Goals annually. These goals are developed based on incidents that have caused severe harm, loss of limb, or death (JCAHO, 2006).

Laser Safety

The introduction of lasers into the surgical arena many years ago provided opportunities for advanced surgical interventions. There are significant safety considerations involved in the use of lasers. The perioperative nurse must be aware of these safety concerns and practice appropriately. The intraoperative phase presents the most vulnerable time for laser-related injury to both patients and personnel if precautions are not followed. The use of lasers presents no concern for the patient when the perioperative nurse follows proper safety precautions.

Lasers come in a variety of wavelengths, depending on the purpose of the laser. The safety measures required for various lasers differ, because lasers display different characteristics and tissue effects related to varying wavelengths. Most lasers require the use of eye protection and some basic safety precautions. The American National Standards Institute (ANSI) provides guidance statements on the safe use of class 3 and class 4 lasers in health care (ANSI, 1996). A laser safety officer should be in place in any health care facility using lasers; this person has the responsibility for ensuring safe laser policies and practices. The perioperative nurse must understand the laser and its use. The nurse monitors the surgical suite for proper signage and ensures that those in the room follow proper procedures, including proper safety measures.

Fire Safety

Operating room fires occur infrequently, but when they do, serious injury or death can result. Knowledge of fire safety is one of the perioperative nurse's responsibilities to ensure safe patient care during the intraoperative phase.

A fire requires three elements that are commonly referred

to as the fire triangle: fuel, ignition, and oxidizer (ECRI, 2006). Fuel is any element that is flammable and can cause a fire, such as sheets, blankets, pillows, drapes, towels, dressings, surgical gowns, and patient gowns. Other items include oxygen masks and tubing, endotracheal tubes, and blood pressure cuffs. Body hair, tissue, and intestinal gas are also considered fuel. Vapors from volatile organic chemicals such as alcohol and acetone are commonly found fuel sources in the operating suite.

The second element in the fire triangle is ignition. Any source of sparking or heat can provide an ignition source. Ignition sources can include surgical lasers, electrocautery equipment, electrosurgical equipment, light sources, and cardiac defibrillators.

Finally, an oxidizer must be present to create fire. Any oxygen rich atmosphere acts as an oxidizer. Pure oxygen, nitrous oxide, or room air can act as an oxidizer, and all of these gases are present in the OR.

The perioperative nurse must maintain vigilance to avoid fires. Staff education and regular fire drills are important components in fire safety practices. The use of electrosurgery is common in most surgical procedures, as is the use of oxygen and the other elements in the fire triangle. The proper use of equipment and materials is important in fire prevention. Electrosurgery pencils should always be holstered when not in use. The operating surgeon should always be the individual operating the foot pedal for electrosurgery or lasers. The anesthesia care provider has control over the oxidizers and should be cognizant of the risks during high-risk surgical procedures, such as head and neck surgery. Effective, clear communication among surgical team members is the best method for preventing fires and taking action if one occurs.

Regulating bodies and other organizations, such as JCAHO, National Fire Protection Association (NFPA), ANSI, ECRI (formerly the Emergency Care Research Institute), and AORN, provide guidelines and criteria for the prevention and management of OR fires and education of staff members.

Radiation

Patients and staff members may be exposed to ionizing radiation, such as x-rays and C-arm, during certain surgical procedures. The perioperative nurse must be aware of the safety precautions to be taken for the surgical team and the patient. Personnel use monitoring devices such as a film badge to determine exposure to ionizing radiation. Scrubbed team members should wear protective equipment, including lead aprons, thyroid shields, eyewear, and lead gloves; circulating personnel should move as far away from the radiation source as possible.

The nurse should assess the patient's reproductive status preoperatively, especially in a female patient, any time ionizing radiation is used. The patient is protected intraoperatively using shielding material that is placed over reproductive organs for studies of the abdomen, hips, and upper legs and over the thyroid when doing procedures involving the head, neck, and upper extremities (Rothrock & Smith, 2003). It is not always possible to shield these areas, but as a patient advocate, the perioperative nurse should try to do so when able.

Principles of Positioning

Patient positioning is an important part of the intraoperative care event. Proper positioning allows for accurate surgical site preparation, appropriate draping, and adequate surgical exposure. Safety and prevention of injury is of paramount importance during positioning. The perioperative nurse must have a thorough understanding of anatomy and physiology as well as the surgical procedure being performed in order to facilitate proper positioning. The equipment used for positioning may be as simple as blankets and pillows or as complex as a fracture table or spinal frame. The nurse must be knowledgeable of all positioning equipment being used.

A variety of factors are involved in patient positioning, and the perioperative nurse should make a thorough assessment of the patient before the start of the procedure. This assessment must include skin integrity; range of motion including restrictions or previous injury; age; medical conditions such as diabetes or arthritis; medications; and the presence of joint or vascular prostheses. The goal of positioning is to provide maximum exposure for the surgeon, minimize risk of physiologic responses to positioning, and facilitate physiologic monitoring (Phillips, 2004). The perioperative nurse must develop a plan of care that includes interventions based on the assessment, such as gathering the appropriate positioning devices, consideration of pressure prevention, avoidance of nerve injury, and amount of assistance needed. The weight limits of OR tables and positioning equipment also must be considered.

External pressure related to positioning can be a predisposing factor to pressure ulcer development. When sitting or lying, body weight is borne by the tissues that cover the bony prominences. When external pressure (i.e., pressure between a bony prominence and a support structure) exceeds capillary pressure, the capillary flow is obstructed and circulation is diminished. Adequate blood flow to tissue provides nourishment and removes accumulated metabolic end products from the area. If this capillary flow is interrupted through constant pressure for two hours, cellular destruction and irreversible tissue damage occurs. The smaller the area with the same amount of pressure, the greater the tissue damage (Porth, 1998).

The proper use of pressure reduction devices is imperative for safe positioning. These may include pressure reduction mattresses, gel pads in many different configurations, pillows, egg crate pads, and donuts for positioning the head. The perioperative nurse must monitor the positioning process to ensure all bony prominences are padded and pressure is distributed evenly. The nurse also must be aware of body alignment and over extension or flexion of joints to prevent stretching of nerves or compression injuries. Proper monitoring of the patient during positioning is an extremely important role for the perioperative nurse.

Monitor and Intervene to Optimize Behavioral Responses of Patient and Family

Health Assessment Techniques; Interviewing Techniques; Communication Theories and Techniques; Behavioral Responses to the Surgical Procedure

From the first encounter between the patient and the perioperative nurse, the nurse seeks to build a relationship based on trust. Using knowledge of psychologist and theorist Maslow's (1908-1970) concept of a hierarchy of needs, and recognizing identified reactions to illness, the perioperative nurse constructs an individualized care plan based on observations of the patient's behavior. The nurse must be sensitive to the patient's verbal and nonverbal messages. Undergoing a surgical procedure is a real threat to the patient's equilibrium and sense of security. A basic fact of behavior holds that a person's psychosocial and physical behavior in response to external stimuli is based on an attempt to maintain homeostasis (Phillips, 2004).

Adaptation to a perceived threat occurs through the use of defense mechanisms. In addition to the physiologic threat, surgical intervention affects the patient's need for security and safety, self-image, and self-actualization. The nurse plans care to address each of these patient needs. Coping mechanisms to counter anxiety are varied. One patient may become withdrawn and uncommunicative, while another talks incessantly or giggles inappropriately. Yet another patient may verbalize anger and impatience. All of these behaviors are identified reactions to stress. The perioperative nurse's goals during this period include careful interpretation of these behavioral messages and implementation of actions to allay anxiety. In planning care of the patient, the nurse recognizes and addresses the patient's need for stress-relieving measures.

Stress can affect both physiologic and psychological function. Physiologically, unrelieved stress can alter digestive, metabolic, wound healing, and autoimmune processes (Phillips, 2004). For many patients, information about the procedure and the sequence of events that are about to occur provides a sense of control in an otherwise frightening and foreign environment. Other patients may request to be told nothing about the surgical procedure. The experienced perioperative nurse understands that coping mechanisms differ greatly among individuals, and are based on factors such as learned patterns, family dynamics, and physiologic status. Providing needed information, speaking slowly while maintaining eye contact, offering reassurance through the use of touch, protecting patient privacy, and limiting external noise and intrusion are all methods the nurse can employ to convey care and concern for the patient's dignity. Surveys indicate that surgical patients desire and expect the perioperative nurse to remain in close physical proximity to them during entry into the OR and induction of anesthesia (Phillips, 2004). The perioperative nurse is the primary protector and advocate for the patient throughout the surgical intervention.

Transcultural Nursing Theory; Theories and Resources for Patient/Family Education; Explications for Perioperative Nurses; Pain Management

A multitude of factors affects the perceptions and behaviors of a patient undergoing surgical intervention. Culture, environment, social and economic status, and family dynamics are all major influences and have to be considered when planning care and detailing desired outcomes. The perioperative nurse plans and delivers care cognizant of the individual's lifestyle, value system, and religious preferences (AORN, 2006).

Patients often make choices regarding their health care based on deeply held beliefs and practices. Religious, social, and cultural factors may predict or dictate the patient's behaviors and responses. Jehovah's Witnesses, for example, will not allow transfusion of blood or blood components, even in life-threatening situations. Other religions, such as Orthodox Jews, mandate observation of dietary restrictions. Still other religions demand modesty in dress and deference to male authority figures. Some cultures expect members to display stoicism and denial in response to pain, while others view loud and emotional reactions as an appropriate response to injury.

The nurse treats the patient with deference and respect for the individual's dignity, beliefs, and personal rights. It is essential that the perioperative nurse identify such social and cultural factors before the surgical intervention. Because these components of the patient's needs pose unique risks and can affect both intraoperative and postoperative outcomes, the plan of care should reflect interventions designed to consider individualized, alternative responses to the identified risks.

Thus, a patient who has a need to suffer pain with stoicism can be observed more closely for nonverbal cues that might indicate the need for pain medication. Surgical technique alterations and careful attention to fluid management and replacement can be employed in the care of the patient who will not allow blood replacement. Necessary exposure can be minimized and delayed until after the patient with rigid modesty is anesthetized. In these ways, the perioperative nurse demonstrates recognition and respect for the dignity and worth of the individual patient, and responds by using critical thinking to adapt the plan of care.

Nursing responsibility includes care for both the patient and the family. Family dynamics can influence the patient experience in a positive or negative fashion. The patient who arrives in the pre-surgical area with a supportive, interested family hovering nearby is probably reassured and comforted by their presence. In other instances, the behavior of family members can serve to further upset an already emotionally stressed patient. The nurse observes and analyzes the interaction of family and patient and employs techniques designed to promote a calm and comforting environment.

Families need information about the progress of their family member during the surgical procedure. Time is perceived to pass more slowly when fear and apprehension are present. Communicating information to the family before, during, and after the surgical procedure gives families a sense of control over the situation and can allay much of the anxiety experienced while waiting. It is essential for families to know what to expect in terms of postoperative care of the patient at home. The perioperative nurse provides necessary information to the family to allow them to properly prepare to care for the family member at home.

Prepare the Surgical Site

The goal of preoperative skin preparation is to reduce the incidence of postoperative surgical site infection. The perioperative nurse is ultimately responsible for ensuring proper preparation of the surgical site. Both the verification of the area to be prepared and the actual physical preparation of the site involve multiple physiologic and safety issues. The nurse implements protective measures to prevent injury due to chemical burn, allergic or toxic reaction, and infection. The perioperative nurse's knowledge of all factors affecting the rationale and actions involved in site preparation is essential to providing safe care and promoting positive patient outcomes.

Preoperative Patient Preparation Activities

Patients may arrive in the surgical area having already showered or otherwise cleansed the surgical site area per preoperative surgeon instruction. Trauma and other emergent cases often necessitate cleansing the operative site area within the OR suite. Regardless of the situation, the skin around the surgical site and surrounding areas should be clean and free of soil or debris prior to the surgical prep. Removal of superficial soil and transient microbes reduces the possibility of wound contamination (AORN, 2006).

Research suggests that, when possible, hair should be left at the surgical site. If necessary, hair removal per preoperative physician order may be performed by mechanical or depilatory method. The affected area should be carefully examined for evidence of skin reaction. Rashes, abrasions, and other insults to skin integrity can provide a means of entry for microorganisms. Adverse skin reactions should be reported to the surgeon, as a severe reaction may result in cancellation of the scheduled procedure.

Anatomy and Physiology; Surgical Procedure

Surgical site preparation requires an in-depth knowledge of anatomic structure and surgical techniques. The perioperative nurse determines the area or areas to be prepared using an understanding of surgical procedures, positioning principles, incision options, and surgeon preferences. Trauma or dual procedure interventions may require preparation of two or more sites at the same time to allow surgeons to operate concurrently. Traumatically injured patients may arrive in the OR with wounds that present challenging surgical site preparation dilemmas. Using knowledge and logic, the nurse adapts the timing and manner of surgical site preparation to provide safe care to the patient and necessary access for the surgical team.

Patient Safety; Principles of Patient's Rights

Surgical site verification is a major patient safety issue for the perioperative team. The RN verbally verifies the site or sites with the identified patient, the operative consent, the surgery schedule, and the surgical team, following institutional policy and recommended practices.

Unnecessary exposure of the patient's body is contrary to the surgical patient's right to privacy, and to the nurse's responsibility to maintain an intraoperative environment conducive to patient dignity. In preparing the patient for surgical site preparation, the nurse demonstrates respect for patient dignity by limiting exposure to only those areas necessary to allow placement of intraoperative monitoring devices and surgical access.

Antiseptic agents used in site preparation should be chosen carefully with consideration for the patient's condition (e.g., intact versus non-intact skin, allergies or sensitivities, and the area to be prepped). A thorough review of the patient's history and previous surgical experience is an invaluable tool for providing information related to prior adverse events. An allergic reaction to a prep solution, resulting in blisters or a rash, may adversely affect the patient outcome. Certain antiseptic agents are contraindicated for use on mucous membranes, while other solutions may be neurotoxic or harmful to pregnant women or neonates. Other safety concerns relative to surgical site preparation include allowing sufficient contact time for the applied antiseptic to be effective and ensuring that alcohol-based solutions are completely evaporated to minimize the risk of fire. Pooling of prep solutions beneath the patient can result in skin breakdown or chemical burns, as well as present a fire hazard in the presence of laser and electrical equipment (AORN, 2006).

Two examples of outcome statements related to the nursing interventions implemented to prevent harm are "The patient is free of signs and symptoms of physical injury" and "The patient is free from signs and symptoms of electrical or laser injury" (Kleinbeck, 2005).

Aseptic Technique; Nursing Research and Evidence-Based Practice; Microbiology and Infection Control

By definition, the surgical incision breaches one of the body's main protective barriers—the skin. Interference with the survival of microorganisms present on the skin around the surgical site can minimize the risk of postoperative wound infection. According to the CDC, up to 16% of all health care-associated infections are surgical site infections (SSI). A majority of the resulting deaths are associated with sepsis related to surgical site infection (Phillips, 2004).

The term "aseptic" refers to the absence of the organisms that cause infection. Techniques and practices to promote surgical asepsis are a focus of the intraoperative plan of care. All actions of the perioperative nurse in performing the surgical prep are directed toward infection prevention.

In assessing the area to be prepped, the nurse employs knowledge of aseptic technique principles and evidence-based practices. Leaving hair at the surgical site is recommended when possible. If removal of hair is required, it should be accomplished outside the OR and as close to the time of surgery as possible. Loose hair has the potential to cause contamination of the surgical wound. Clippers have been shown to be the least irritating method of hair removal. Razors and depilatories can cause abrasion and irritation of the skin, predisposing the area to bacterial colonization (AORN, 2006).

In determining the area to be prepared, the nurse should consider the possibilities for additional procedures or extended incisions. Sterile supplies are used to perform the prep. An antiseptic is chosen based on recommended practices, surgeon preference, and range of germicidal activity. Burned or traumatized skin should be prepped with a nonirritating solution, such as normal saline. The perioperative nurse demonstrates understanding that friction is the primary mechanism by which bacteria are removed from the surgical site. Areas of high microbial content must be isolated from cleaner areas and prepped last. Skin preparation proceeds from the site of the incision to the outer margin of the area being prepared. The prepared area is allowed to dry before application of surgical draping material.

Documentation of All Nursing Interventions

Thorough documentation of all actions taken by the perioperative nurse in preparing the surgical site is important to communication and the flow of information between care providers. Condition of the skin both before and after skin preparation should be noted. In addition, all documentation should include the area prepared, the prepping agent, the person performing the prep, and any adverse skin or systemic reactions related to the prepping agent. The method of hair removal should be noted if applicable. Data collected from documentation of surgical skin preparation techniques, agents, and adverse reactions contribute to evaluation of current practices and promotes improvement of patient outcomes.

Select Procedure-Specific Protective Barrier Materials

Principles of Product Evaluation and Cost Containment

Surgical procedures require the use of gowns and drapes to ensure a sterile field for preventing contamination and infection of the surgical site. Surgical gowns also provide a barrier to protect the scrubbed personnel from exposure to blood borne pathogens. Materials may be disposable or reusable, and selection is based on desired effect, comfort, and amount of projected exposure. Guidelines are available to assist the perioperative nurse in the selection of barrier materials to ensure adequate protection for the desired purpose.

The AORN Recommended Practices for Selection and Use of Surgical Gowns and Drapes advise that materials used for gowns and drapes should be resistant to penetration by blood or body fluids (AORN, 2006). The projected purpose and risk for exposure should be considered when selecting the barrier material required. AORN further recommends that those involved in the purchasing decision evaluate the products based on manufacturers' data indicating amount of protection against fluids, particulates, and transfer of microorganisms. Material also should be puncture and tear resistant to avoid contamination. Other considerations include the material's ability to be sterilized using appropriate methods, resistance to combustion, comfort, and cost-benefit ratio. When deciding on a gown or drape, the cost should not be the only area of consideration. While cost is definitely important, the value and performance of the product also must be evaluated.

The perioperative nurse has an important role in ensuring appropriate selection of barrier materials. While the nurse may not be involved in the negotiation or final purchasing decision, participation in trials and providing feedback are very important elements in the selection of appropriate barrier materials.

Monitor and Evaluate the Effects of Anesthetic Agents

The perioperative nurse's role and responsibility related to anesthetic management of the intraoperative patient varies in scope, depending upon the presence of an anesthesia care provider, the health status of the patient, and the anesthetic technique employed. In unison with the surgical team, the RN supports a coordinated effort to ensure a safe and effective anesthesia experience for the patient.

Pathophysiology; Physiology Responses to the Surgical Experience Including Potential Complications

Chapter 7 provides an in-depth discussion of the physiologic mechanisms and actions of general versus local anesthetic methods and agents and describes American Society of Anesthesiologists (ASA) risk classification, varying levels of sedation, and appropriate responses to cardiac arrest and malignant hyperthermia emergencies.

The perioperative RN has clearly defined professional responsibilities related to specific types of anesthesia. Local or moderate sedation techniques require the presence of a dedicated nurse, with no competing responsibilities, to monitor the patient, administer medications, interpret data and responses, and intervene to prevent complications. The nurse should demonstrate current knowledge of commonly used medications and systemic effects, as well as ability to recognize signs and symptoms of toxic or allergic reactions. Patients who are determined to be too sick to permit general anesthesia are not appropriate candidates for local anesthesia without the presence of an anesthesia care provider (Phillips, 2004), and institutional and anesthesia department policies should address these issues.

The nurse monitoring the patient undergoing local or moderate sedation procedures should follow specific institutional policies defining the role of the nurse during these types of anesthetic interventions. At a minimum, policies should require monitoring of pulse, blood pressure, oxygen saturation, and respiration. Policies guided by AORN recommended practices promote evidence-based, high level care for the surgical patient. The perioperative nurse establishes baseline vital signs and observes for changes in physiologic data related to the surgical intervention and administration of pharmacologic agents. In most instances, the monitoring RN functions under the direction of the physician performing the surgical procedure and reports responses and adverse reactions directly to the surgeon. The nurse is responsible for accurate documentation of all pertinent data relative to medication administration, physiologic monitoring, and patient responses. Documentation of all relative data is important to the understanding and evaluation of patient outcomes.

Anesthetic Interventions (e.g., assist as needed)

The primary role of the perioperative RN in the delivery of regional and general anesthetics is to assist the anesthesia care provider with all appropriate and required interventions. Before entering the surgical suite, the nurse reviews the patient medical record, noting the history and physical, presence of allergies, and any abnormal or missing lab data. This information and any other pertinent facts are shared with the anesthesia care provider to provide a consistent and coordinated plan of care.

Depending on institution policy, some regional nerve blocks are initiated in the holding or receiving area of surgery. Nursing care includes aiding in exposure of the injection site, providing for the privacy and modesty of the patient, and offering emotional support during the procedure.

A Bier block is a regional anesthetic technique that requires placement of a double-cuffed tourniquet to the proximal portion of the extremity. The RN assists with tourniquet placement and the subsequent elevation and exsanguination of the operative extremity.

Spinal and general anesthetic techniques require the perioperative nurse to facilitate positioning and assist in maintenance of the patient in either a lateral or sitting position. The professional nurse provides support to the patient and monitors maintenance of aseptic technique at the injection site.

General anesthesia requires the presence of the nurse during induction, maintenance, and emergence from anesthesia. During induction and emergence, controlling environmental noise and room traffic can greatly reduce patient anxiety. As a patient advocate, the nurse understands the psychological importance of being physically present with the patient through the induction phase. Equally important during this time is the nurse's ability to aid in such actions as transferring the patient, providing warmth, obtaining intravenous access, and placing monitoring devices.

Placement of prophylactic antiembolic devices, such as compression stockings or sequential compression sleeves powered by a motorized pump, should be initiated before induction. General anesthesia reduces venous return and causes vasodilatation, which may precipitate formation of deep venous thrombosis (DVT) and pulmonary emboli (Phillips, 2004).

During intubation, the RN may be asked to provide cricoid pressure to prevent regurgitation of stomach contents and aid in visualization of the airway. Known as Sellick's maneuver, this manual compression of the esophagus is not released until successful intubation has been verified, the cuff inflated, and the tube secured by the anesthesia care provider.

Positioning the surgical patient is done only after permission to proceed is given by the anesthesia care provider. The perioperative nurse facilitates anatomic positioning to prevent nerve or tissue damage due to pressure or stretching. Appropriate warming devices are initiated and maintained. The perioperative RN monitors physiologic responses of the patient, cooperates with the anesthesia care provider in calculation of blood loss, and assists with fluid and volume replacement interventions.

During emergence from anesthesia, the endotracheal tube is maintained until the recovery of pharyngeal and laryngeal reflexes and the return of spontaneous respiration (Phillips, 2004).

At the end of the procedure, report is communicated to the receiving unit (e.g., PACU or intensive care unit) to ensure adequate preparation and transfer of vital information. Some essential elements of the postoperative report include the estimated time of arrival in the unit, surgical procedure, anesthesia method, physiologic condition, blood and fluid replacement, special positioning requirements, ventilator status, and/or mechanical ventilation settings. The perioperative nurse consults with the anesthesia care provider for specific information to be relayed in the report.

In the joint operative effort between anesthesia and perioperative professionals, the nurse demonstrates an ability to coordinate and manage all interactions of the multidisciplinary surgical team. Interventions that provide safe, competent, and patient-centric care promote and maintain the integrity and trust inherent in the patient-nurse relationship.

Monitor and Evaluate the Effects of Pharmacologic Agents

Commitment to patient safety demands that the perioperative nurse demonstrate current knowledge and understanding of intended use, sterile application, proper dosage, and adverse effects of all chemicals, drugs, and mixtures used in intraoperative care. Dispensing and mixing of such pharmaceutical substances require strict attention to details of sterile technique and medication management.

Pharmacology and Anesthetic Agents; Principles of Patient Safety

Pharmaceutical applications relative to anesthetic interventions are discussed in a previous section. Surgical pharmacology refers to more than just medications. Substances used during surgical intervention can be derived from a vast array of both biologic and synthetic sources. Joint prosthetics and other types of implants constitute permanent changes to the body, while other materials may be systematically absorbed over time. Many drugs are designed specifically for use in the OR. Pharmacologic strategies use agents in solid, liquid, powder, and gaseous states. Preparations such as dyes, surgical incision adhesives, tissue stains, contrast media, hemostatic coagulants, tumescence solutions, and gaseous materials are but a few examples of the pharmacologic agents manufactured for specialty use in the surgical environment (Phillips, 2004).

The perioperative nurse implements a plan of care to protect the patient from harm. Every action of the surgical team is examined for adherence to principles of patient safety. The nurse has a legal and ethical obligation to demonstrate competency in the handling of all pharmacologic substances used during the intraoperative phase. Competency includes familiarity with both generic and trade names of commonly used medications, knowledge of adverse effects, and adherence to recommended practices related to medication safety.

All pharmaceutical substances introduced to the sterile field should be labeled. Labels should clearly identify the drug name, strength, dosage, and date of expiration if applicable. Institutional policies for labeling should reference the AORN Guidance Statement on Safe Medication Practices in Perioperative Settings Across the Lifespan (AORN, 2006). The five "R"s of medication safety—right patient, right medication, right dose, right time, right route—are employed in all pharmacologic interventions. Instances of uncertainty or unfamiliarity regarding names or dosages of specific medications should be resolved by using available resources. The *Physicians' Desk Reference* (PDR), the anesthesia care provider, the surgeon, or the hospital pharmacist can provide guidance and information about specifics of a particular drug. The surgical patient relies on the skill and knowledge of the surgical team to deliver an optimal outcome.

Pain Management; Physiologic Responses to the Surgical Experience Including Potential Complications

Pharmacologic agents are used intraoperatively both as prophylactics and in response to physiologic changes experienced by the surgical patient. Antibiotics are given to prevent surgical site infections, as well as to treat existing sources of infection. Pain medication is delivered to the patient as a component of balanced anesthetic management and in anticipation of postoperative discomfort. Surgical patients expect adequate pain relief, and discussion of individual attitudes, beliefs, and knowledge relative to postoperative pain control are an important part of the initial perioperative assessment. Patient participation in preoperative planning for appropriate pain management involves realistic goal setting, review of pain relief strategies, and defining patient rights and responsibilities. The perioperative nurse has a professional duty to ensure that the patient receives information and instruction related to postoperative analgesia.

Intraoperatively, requests for surgical pharmaceuticals may be communicated as a written order or a verbal request. Drugs also may be made available for use in response to documented surgeon preferences. Pharmaceutical agents are used to counter and treat physiologic responses related to the stress of the surgical procedure and anesthesia. The nurse assists the anesthesia care provider and the surgical team in monitoring patient responses and obtaining and delivering the necessary pharmacologic substances. Use of any drug is verified verbally with the requesting surgeon or anesthesia care provider before it is dispensed to the sterile field. The circulating nurse and the scrub technician or nurse visually and verbally verify the drug name, concentration, and expiration date during delivery to the field. Any patient allergies are also noted at this time. Techniques for dispensing solutions and other pharmacological materials should be developed by individual facilities and reflect JCAHO standards and AORN recommended practices.

Pharmaceuticals commonly used to diagnose or respond to various physiologic alterations, complications, and anticipated outcomes include:

- antibiotics,
- hemostatic materials,
- anticoagulants,
- anti-anxiety medications,
- thrombolytics,
- local anesthetics,
- surgical dyes and stains,
- analgesics,
- adrenergic agonists,
- antidysrhythmics,
- lubricants, and
- expansion media (Phillips, 2004).

Identify and Control Environmental Factors

Control of the surgical environment is critical for safe procedures. Environmental control consists of many facets, including temperature, humidity, traffic flow, noise, cleaning, hazardous spills, and fires. The perioperative nurse must take responsibility to ensure that proper monitoring takes place and procedures are followed to ensure compliance with regulations and to promote quality care for the patient.

Environmental Factors (temperature, humidity, air exchanges)

The most common organisms found in surgical site infections are *S. epidermidis* and *S. aureus* (Spry, 2005). These microorganisms are typically found on the skin. As the number of people in the operating suite increases, the risk of microorganism shedding and dispersion into the air increases. Motion stirs the air in the room and disperses these microorganisms. As the organisms travel through the air, they can settle into the surgical site where an SSI may develop. To minimize the risk of contamination by these airborne particles, the perioperative nurse should keep the number of personnel and motion in the room to a minimum.

The American Institute of Architects published the "Guidelines for Construction and Equipment of Hospital and Medical Facilities" (AIA, 2001). These guidelines include recommendations for air exchanges, temperature, and humidity levels that facilitate prevention of infection.

Each OR should have a minimum of 15 air exchanges per hour. Three of these replacements should be from outside filtered air (Rothrock, 2003). Air is delivered to the room through ceiling or high wall vents and exhausted through outlets near the floor and on the wall opposite the inflow vents. Drafts should be at a minimum. The OR should be maintained with positive pressure to prevent inflow of less filtered, more contaminated air. Doors must remain closed to prevent pressure equalization.

Humidity should remain between 30% and 60% (Rothrock, 2003). Lower humidity increases the risk of static electricity and sparking, which can be an ignition source for fire. Lower humidity also can result in more dust-carrying bacteria in the environment. Higher humidity may cause condensation on supplies and equipment. This resulting dampness can result in strikethrough contamination of sterile items and can support bacterial growth.

The surgical suite temperature should be maintained between 68° F and 73° F, or 20° C to 23° C (Spry, 2005). This temperature inhibits bacterial growth and provides a comfortable environment for the surgical team. The perioperative nurse is responsible for ensuring that the temperature and humidity are within acceptable ranges. This should be recorded daily.

To avoid increased risk of airborne contamination, the nurse should plan activities to avoid unnecessary travel in and out of the surgical suite. This includes anticipating surgeon needs and having equipment, supplies, and instruments readily available in the room. The nurse also should keep personnel and motion in the room to a minimum to decrease the number of airborne bacteria shed from individuals. The circulating nurse must remain vigilant during the intraoperative phase to advocate infection prevention for the patient.

Noise

Noise can be present in many forms. Music, instruments such as drills and saws, shuffling paper, talking, suction, monitoring equipment, and clattering of instruments touching can all be sources of noise. Noise can be distracting or irritating to the surgeon and the surgical team, resulting in decreased concentration and efficiency or missed communication of important information. The patient is very sensitive to sound during induction of general anesthesia and aware of conversations and other sounds during local anesthesia or light sedation.

Music should be low and soothing if played while the patient can hear it. It should never interfere with any member of the surgical team's ability to communicate or monitor physiologic functions. Conversations should be quiet and patient-centered. The focus of conversation should be on the patient during induction and emergence from anesthesia. Discussion during this time may be interpreted by the patient as pertaining to him or her directly. Suction can be clamped when not in use and alarms or operating indicators can be turned to low volume.

The perioperative nurse is responsible for monitoring noise levels and minimizing these as much as possible. Conversation and planning between the surgical team members in advance of the procedure can facilitate this. While it may be uncomfortable to do, the nurse has the right and the obligation to request patient focused conversation, that music volume is tolerable to all members of the team, and that other sources of noise are controlled.

Performing Environmental Cleaning (room turnover, spills, terminal cleaning)

Maintaining a clean environment in the OR is paramount to preventing surgical site infections. Room cleaning should start before surgeries begin, be performed between surgical procedures and patients, and completed at the end of the day. Cleaning should be performed using only an EPA-registered hospital-grade germicidal agent. Before the first procedure for the day, all horizontal surfaces including tables, furniture, and surgical lights should be damp dusted using a cloth dampened with germicidal agent. Dust that accumulates overnight may become a vector for microorganisms. Any equipment coming from another area must be cleaned before being brought into the OR from outside. The perioperative nurse should verify that the surgical suite has been prepared and cleaned properly before the first case of the day and between each case. As a patient advocate, the perioperative nurse has a responsibility to ensure a safe environment for each patient.

Room Turnover:
Cleaning is important during room turnover to remove potential contaminants and to prepare the room for the next patient. Any items that contact the patient or surgical site are considered contaminated (Spry, 2005). Personnel should wear personal protective equipment, including gloves and eye shields, when performing room turnover. All disposable items should be discarded in the appropriate containers. Infectious waste is placed in biohazard labeled waste containers; rigid plastic containers must be used for any sharp objects such as needles, scalpel blades, and staples.

Liquid waste is disposed of in the hopper, solidified using an agent designed for this purpose, or in a liquid waste disposal system. Solidified liquid waste is disposed of in the appropriate biohazard container. Instruments are removed from the OR covered or in closed containers and taken to the decontamination area where they are cleaned and prepared for sterilization. Linens should be placed into linen bags, taking care to avoid shaking or dragging. All equipment that contacts the patient should be cleaned using a germicidal agent. Walls, doors, and surgical lights should be spot cleaned if spattered with blood, tissue, or body fluids. Floors that are visibly soiled should be mopped using a clean mop head dipped into a germicidal solution (AORN, 2006).

Spills:
Spills may occur at any time and are a source for potential injury if not cleaned up immediately and properly. Small spills of body fluid or blood should be cleaned immediately using an absorbent lint-free cloth followed by application of a germicidal agent, leaving it on the surface for the

time specified for the agent (AORN, 2006). Large spills (over 10 mL) should be treated using a disposable absorbent material and followed with a germicidal agent.

Terminal Cleaning:
At the end of the day, equipment and areas of the OR should be terminally cleaned. This terminal cleaning reduces the number of microorganisms, dust, and organic debris in the surgical environment and lowers the risk of contamination and infection. The areas requiring terminal cleaning include:

- surgical lights and tracks,
- ceiling-mounted or fixed equipment,
- all equipment and furniture,
- hallways and floors,
- handles on cabinets and push plates on walls,
- ventilation grills,
- all horizontal surfaces (e.g., counter tops, shelving),
- substerile areas,
- scrub and utility areas, and
- scrub sinks.

These items should be cleaned using an EPA-registered germicidal agent and mechanical friction. The OR floors should be wet-vacuumed using a hospital-grade disinfectant at least once in a 24-hour period (AORN, 2006).

Maintain a Sterile Field Including Aseptic Technique

The perioperative nurse has a primary responsibility to protect the patient from infection. Maintenance of the sterile field during surgical intervention requires diligence and a joint cooperative effort by the entire surgical team. Knowledge of microbiology and a thorough understanding of the principles of surgical asepsis are necessary components of the intraoperative plan of care.

Surgical Procedure; Aseptic Technique

During the intraoperative phase, careful monitoring of aseptic practices is required of both scrubbed and unscrubbed personnel. All scrubbed personnel function within the confines of the established sterile field and should be garbed according to recommended practices. This attire includes scrub clothing, sterile gowns and gloves, caps, masks, and protective eyewear. The purpose of surgical attire is twofold. It protects the patient from transfer of microorganisms to the surgical site, thus reducing the possibility of surgical site infection; it also reduces the exposure of OR personnel to bloodborne disease and infectious organisms (AORN, 2006).

Following evidence-based practices, a sterile field should be prepared for every patient, regardless of the type of procedure or the presence of existing infection. All items used within the sterile field should be sterile, and sterile drapes are used to delineate the boundaries of the surgical field. Surgical drapes should not be repositioned after placement, as this movement may facilitate transfer of microorganisms to the surgical site (AORN, 2006).

Unscrubbed personnel responsible for transfer of items to the sterile field should follow practices designed to maintain the integrity of the field. All items delivered to the sterile field should be inspected for package integrity, external indication of sterility, and expiration date. There is no "degree" of sterility. An item is either sterile or not sterile. If questions exist as to an item's sterility, the item in question is either discarded or unwrapped and resterilized. As discussed in an earlier section, factors related to traffic and noise control, room temperature and humidity, and cleanliness and condition of room equipment, affect the quality and preservation of the sterile field. Control of these environmental circumstances is integral to providing a safe environment and promoting desired patient outcomes.

The circulating nurse bears ultimate responsibility for optimizing and safeguarding the environment in which surgical intervention takes place. All surgical personnel have a duty to monitor, recognize, report, and correct breaks in sterile field maintenance. A single break in technique can irreparably harm the patient, whose health and life are entrusted to the care of the surgical team (Phillips, 2004). The term "surgical conscience" suggests a personal acknowledgement of this individual, professional responsibility.

The PNDS describes a desired outcome related to aseptic technique maintenance. Outcome 010, "the patient is free from signs and symptoms of infection," falls under the physiologic domain in the PNDS nomenclature, and is further defined as the patient being free from other signs and symptoms of health care-acquired infection such as pain, odor, drainage, or fever within a 30-day period subsequent to the surgical intervention (Kleinbeck, 2005).

Principles of Wound Healing; Microbiology and Infection Control

Because surgical interventions, by design and definition, breach protective barriers to pathogenic invasion, every surgical patient has a potential risk for infection. All surgical aseptic practice is guided by acknowledgement of this inherent threat to patient safety.

Specific phases of wound healing are discussed in an earlier section. Surgical wound healing is affected by a multitude of factors. Patients undergoing surgical procedures may have pre-existing physiologic conditions that compromise healing. Co-existing morbidities such as diabetes, vascular disease, resistant bacterial infections, or immune disorders can greatly influence the mechanism of wound healing. A patient arriving in the operative arena with an open, grossly contaminated wound is already at high risk for postoperative complications related to wound infection. Most surgical site infections are related to contamination of the sterile field by the surgical team. A localized surgical site infection can quickly become a systemic sepsis that threatens the health and life of the patient (Phillips, 2004).

The body protects itself from disease with intact systems of defense. The first line of defense is the skin and mucous membranes as barriers to pathogenic invasion. The second line of defense involves an inflammatory response to an insult or injury to first line defenses. Passive or actively acquired immunity is the body's third line of defense in the battle against infectious organisms. Understanding how various pathogens are transmitted, the conditions in which they proliferate, and effective methods for causing microbial death, is essential to preventing surgical site infections.

As knowledge evolves regarding antibiotic selection and timing, maintenance of perioperative normothermia, glucose level control, and other intraoperative variables, infection prevention protocols will change to reflect current evidence and best practices. The perioperative nurse's assessment of potential for infection combines knowledge of microbiology, understanding of infection control principles, and ongoing education. Flexibility and the ability to apply critical thinking skills to adapt to a given situation are attributes essential to effective intraoperative nursing practice.

Principles of Sterilization and Disinfection; Disinfection Procedures for Equipment and Instruments

Maintaining the uncompromised sterility of the operative field is essential to the safety of the patient. Because every patient is also a potential source of infection for the health care team, all instruments used during the surgical procedure are terminally decontaminated and sterilized after completion of the case. The scrub person initiates the decontamination process by wiping instruments as they are used during the surgical intervention. Decontamination is a combination of mechanical and chemical cleaning processes (Phillips, 2004). Initial decontamination of both instruments and equipment is performed according to facility policy and recommended practices.

In many settings, a central service department has responsibility for decontamination, disinfection, and sterilization of all surgical instruments. In other health care institutions, surgical staff may be required to perform decontamination, disinfection, and sterilization procedures in a designated room outside the OR. Safety methods must be employed to protect the health care worker from occupational exposure during processing of instruments and terminal cleaning of equipment.

Methods of disinfection include manual wiping with a chemical disinfectant, immersion and soaking, and specialized machinery to flush contaminants from instrument surfaces (Phillips, 2004). Sterilization methods appropriate to the item being sterilized are implemented according to recommended practices for sterilization. Chapter 6 discusses specific characteristics, methods, and regulatory requirements related to the cleaning, disinfection, and sterilization of surgical instruments.

Test and Use Equipment According to Manufacturers' Recommendations

Instruments, Supplies, and Equipment Relating to Surgical Procedure

Technology is evident in many areas of health care, but especially in the surgical arena. The perioperative nurse may be responsible for numerous pieces of equipment in the OR, depending on the procedure being performed. The nurse must demonstrate competence with each piece of equipment to ensure a problem-free surgery and positive outcomes for the patient.

Criteria for measuring competency may include:

- list standard components to a particular system (e.g., video);
- describe the function of components or piece of equipment;
- demonstrate operation of the equipment;
- choose appropriate items to use with the equipment (e.g., electrosurgery adapter, suction connecter);
- locate equipment alarms and explain their purpose; and
- identify safety precautions required for the equipment.

Any person responsible for medical equipment used in the OR should be properly instructed on all aspects of it before use and periodically to maintain competency.

Principles of Equipment Inspection and Maintenance

Any new piece of equipment brought into the hospital should have an incoming inspection to test for electrical safety. A member of the clinical engineering department completes this inspection. The biomedical or clinical engineering technician is a valuable member of the perioperative team who helps maintain and troubleshoot any patient care equipment in the health care facility. Some hospitals have a dedicated biomedical engineering technician for the OR. Equipment is scheduled for inspection at specific time intervals by the biomedical technician to ensure proper functioning and continued safety of the device. Each piece of equipment should have a sticker identifying that it has been checked and approved for use by the clinical engineering department. The perioperative nurse ensures that all equipment used has this sticker in place.

It is the perioperative nurse's responsibility to report any equipment problems or malfunctions to the clinical engineering department. Before using any equipment, it should be inspected for frayed or cut electrical cords, loose connections, damaged or missing controls, damaged foot pedals or connecting cords, or malfunctioning alarms. Any malfunctioning or broken equipment should be removed from service and reported to the clinical engineering department immediately. Following these practices promotes patient and staff safety.

Practices and Guidelines: Organizations

The Association for the Advancement of Medical Instrumentation (AAMI) was founded in 1967 with a goal of increasing the understanding and beneficial use of medical instrumentation. It is a valuable source of timely information on medical instrumentation and technology and provides the standards that are followed by industry, professions, and the government for safe and effective use of medical instrumentation (AAMI, 2006).

ECRI (formerly the Emergency Care Research Institute) is a non-profit health services research agency with a mission to improve the safety, quality, and cost-effectiveness of health care (ECRI, 2006). It is designated as an Evidence-based Practice Center (EPC) by the U. S. Agency for Healthcare Research and Quality. ECRI provides alerts regarding health care system and technology-related hazards and includes strategies to correct them. They also share medical product evaluations and health technology assessments.

The information that these agencies provide is a valuable tool for the perioperative nurse and the clinical engineering professional in the selection and operation of surgical equipment.

Maintain the Dignity, Modesty, and Privacy of the Patient

During the intraoperative phase, the perioperative nurse acts as guardian of the patient's dignity and unique nature and also shows respect for individual cultural and spiritual concerns. The patient is responsible for providing accurate information to the caregiver. In understanding and consenting to surgical intervention, the patient enters into an ethical and legal agreement, and forms an unspoken and sacred bond with the surgical team.

Patient Rights and Responsibilities; Regulatory Standards and Voluntary Guidelines (ANA Code of Ethics, AORN Standards, Recommended Practices and Guidelines)

All patients have a right to participate in decisions affecting their own care. Once the decision to proceed with surgical intervention has been made, the surgical patient may feel stripped of control regarding the surgical event. Surgical intervention constitutes an invasion of the human body. In the view of the patient, surgery involves a loss of dignity, and many required interventions appear impersonal and threatening to individuality.

When observed from the perspective of the surgical patient, the events occurring in the course of surgical intervention are strange and frightening.

- Personnel stand in a dominant position, looking down on a patient lying supine on a bed.
- Glasses and teeth are removed, limiting vision and affecting speech and appearance.
- Hair is covered by a "one size fits all" cap.
- Personal clothing is removed and replaced with standard patient garb not known for preserving modesty.
- Consciousness and the ability to reason are altered.

The American Nurses Association (ANA) *Code of Ethics* requires that nurses practice with respect for "the inherent dignity, worth, and uniqueness" of each patient (ANA, 2001). The perioperative nurse recognizes that maintaining an environment respectful of individuality and dignity is essential to reducing patient anxiety and optimizing outcomes. The nurse exercises proper decorum during introduction and interview. The patient is consulted as to preferences and is allowed to make simple choices when possible (e.g., intravenous [IV] line in the right or left arm, family present or sent to the waiting room). Proper names are used during conversation; use of nicknames or first names is avoided unless preferred by the patient. The perioperative RN allows for questions and answers in a manner that preserves patient privacy. Eye contact and active listening enhance the nurse's effort to create a relationship of trust with the patient. Actions are explained before physical contact and touching occur. In all of these ways, the nurse demonstrates concern and recognition for the patient's sense of self.

Environmental Factors; Principles of Positioning

The perioperative nurse monitors and controls many factors that affect care of the surgical patient. Controlling personnel traffic aids in ensuring patient privacy and reduces the risk of infection. Limiting extraneous noise and unnecessary conversation in the operating suite promotes an environment conducive to reducing anxiety. Minimizing exposure during placement of monitors and providing for warmth enhances patient comfort and maintenance of dignity. Issues related to concerns about exposure are communicated to the surgical team. The perioperative professional nurse designs interventions to promote an atmosphere of privacy and concern for the patient. Anti-embolism stockings can be applied in a manner consistent with preservation of modesty, and actions such as tourniquet placement can be delayed until after induction.

Patients undergoing regional or local anesthetics are often awake and aware of exposure required by interventions such as Foley catheter placement, prepping, and positioning. Explaining actions and providing a privacy drape or curtain to shield the patient's view of these activities demonstrates consideration for the patient's sense of modesty. During positioning, care is planned to provide adequate access to the surgical site while minimizing unnecessary bodily exposure. Operating room personnel should be diligent in ensuring that all conversations reflect professional attitudes and behaviors.

The perioperative RN bears ultimate responsibility for maintenance of an intraoperative environment that ensures protection of patient dignity. The nurse demonstrates depth of knowledge in regard to the ethical responsibility to safeguard the surgical patient from both real and perceived threats to personal dignity and personhood. The perspective of each individual patient is unique and meaningful. The nurse honors a commitment to treat the patient with respect for individual behaviors and beliefs.

Protect Patient Confidentiality

The handling of personal health information is strictly defined and regulated. In the intraoperative setting, the RN is guided by ethical principles, follows governmental and regulatory statutes, and implements specific institutional policies designed to maintain the privacy of protected personal health information.

Legal Responsibilities

According to the Health Insurance Portability and Accountability Act (HIPAA) of 1996, parties who deal with personal health information must exercise reasonable caution in the collection, storage, and transmission of such information (US Department of HHS, 2006). Both governmental and regulatory agencies monitor health care providers' compliance with established policies and procedures for the handling and maintenance of private patient information. Protected health information is generally understood to include all information that could identify a particular patient. Institutional bodies are mandated to establish methods to strictly control the flow and maintenance of such data. All health care organizations require employees to be knowledgeable and demonstrate legal and ethical competency in regard to the management of private health information.

Interviewing Techniques; Surgical Consent Process

All patients expect privacy. The perioperative RN demonstrates knowledge of HIPAA regulations and honors the confidentiality of personal health information in planning interventions to care for the surgical patient. In the intraoperative setting, attention to multiple situational factors is necessary to protect patient information. Some examples include:

- providing a private environment for the patient interview and assessment;
- determining the patient's wishes regarding presence of family members during interview;
- maintaining written or viewable patient information in a controlled area;
- speaking in a tone of voice not audible to surrounding parties; and
- limiting access to intraoperative test results and reports.

In designing a plan of care, the nurse demonstrates a legal and ethical regard for patient confidentiality. The nature of the information exchanged between the surgical patient and the perioperative RN is often highly sensitive and may be difficult or embarrassing for the patient to verbalize. The nurse employs therapeutic modalities of communication designed to allay anxiety and facilitate the gathering of data relevant to the formation of nursing diagnoses. A patient may verbalize knowledge of the surgical procedure and verify informed consent, yet request to be told no further details about what will occur during the experience. The perioperative nurse plans interventions to address the individual needs of the patient and shows concern for, and adherence to, all measures pertinent to the safeguarding of personal health information.

Advocate For and Protect Patient Rights

The American Hospital Association's (AHA) Patient Bill of Rights defines the health care patient's entitlement to certain basic components of care. Every patient has a right to expect competent, standardized, and nonjudgmental care in any health care setting or situation involved in the delivery of such care (AHA, 2006). The perioperative environment requires specific interventions designed to address issues related to intraoperative events and expected patient outcomes.

Implications for Patient Care; Principles of Patients' Rights

The perioperative nurse champions patient rights by providing competent and ethically sound care to all surgical patients, irrespective of socioeconomic, cultural, or situational factors. Patients arrive in the intraoperative area expecting a successful surgical outcome. After the assessment and formation of nursing diagnoses initiated by the nurse, specific interventions are planned to meet desired goals relative to these expected outcomes. Domain 3B, which deals with behavioral responses of the surgical patient, include the PNDS competency statements relevant to patient rights and address areas of ethical, legal, and moral responsibility (AORN, 2006). The perioperative nurse understands that standards of ethical practice mandate the delivery of non-differential care to every patient.

Barriers to communication, such as language differences or sensory impairment, are addressed with interventions such as the use of an interpreter or family member to facilitate understanding and flow of information. The nurse evaluates the effectiveness of these actions and adjusts the plan of care in response. If the patient expresses a desire to have family members present during the interview process, the RN supports family participation. In providing an environment sensitive to the patient's individual needs, the perioperative nurse ensures that information and interventions are delivered to the patient in a manner conducive to therapeutic response and outcomes.

Principles of Patient Safety; Pain Management

The perioperative RN advocates for the patient using knowledge of risks and prescribed interventions. The patient is at risk for pain related to the surgical intervention, and management of pain is a primary concern. The nurse assesses the current pain status of the patient and evaluates the effectiveness of any current pain relief regimens. Allergies to medications are noted and interventions are designed to control pain throughout the perioperative period. The nurse continually evaluates the effectiveness of pain management interventions and adapts the plan of care in response to the patient's feedback.

The surgical environment also poses many challenges to the maintenance of patient safety. Some examples of specific intraoperative safety measures include:

- verification of informed consent and surgical site;
- protecting the patient from burn hazards associated with use of electrical devices;
- identification of allergic reactions to skin preparation solutions or antibiotics;
- positioning the patient in a manner to avoid tissue or nerve injury;
- shielding the patient from unnecessary radiological exposure;
- maintaining aseptic technique to prevent wound infection;
- following established procedures for maintenance of implanted devices; and
- evaluating responses to planned interventions and adjusting care accordingly.

All care is planned to protect the health and safety of the surgical patient and provide for optimal outcomes. Safeguards initiated by the perioperative nurse are reflective of a commitment to act in a manner consistent with ethical and professional advocacy.

Prepare and Label Specimens

Legal Responsibilities and Implications for Patient Care

Most surgical procedures produce a specimen of some type: tissue, fluid, or foreign body. The perioperative nurse is responsible for ensuring the proper care and handling of specimens, as these factors affect the outcome of surgery. Specimens should be handled as infectious and secured in leak proof containers for transport to pathology, lab, radiology, or other destinations designated by the surgeon.

Clear specimen labeling must be in place and include the specimen name, source, description of any tags placed on the specimen (e.g., "suture at 4 o'clock indicates location of mass"), patient name and other identifier (usually a medical record number), date and time specimen obtained, and surgeon. Labeling should indicate if a report should be called to the surgeon immediately, such as with a frozen section specimen. Specimens should be separated in different containers, especially when sending two of the same type of specimen or sending multiple biopsies.

Some specimens are processed differently as dictated by the testing desired. The perioperative nurse must be aware of the method for handling the specimen including whether the specimen will be placed in solution, such as saline or formalin, or remain dry. The method of preparation is as important as properly labeling and transporting the specimen. The pathology report remains a permanent part of the medical record and provides essential information that guides the surgeon's plan of treatment.

Forensic specimens require special treatment and should follow a chain of custody to ensure the evidence is secure at all times. Follow appropriate hospital policies. These policies should mirror the AORN Recommended Practices for the Care and Handling of Specimens in the Perioperative Environment (AORN, 2006).

Document Intraoperative Activities: Document Specimens and Disposition of the Specimens

Specimen collection and disposition must be entered in the operative procedure record that remains a permanent part of the patient's legal medical record. Include in the documentation the specimen, location, any tags or markings on the specimen, destination, and how it was handled: formalin, saline, dry, fresh or frozen section.

Examples:

3/20/06 Specimen: right tube and ovary in formalin sent to pathology

6/18/06 Specimen: tissue mass right breast with wire intact sent fresh to radiology for examination

9/30/06 Specimen #1: skin lesion, left forearm, in formalin, to pathology
Specimen #2: skin lesion, right upper anterior thigh, in formalin, to pathology

Label Solutions, Medications, and Medication Containers

Regulatory Standards and Voluntary Guidelines

All nurses are responsible for safe medication handling and administration. The use of medications and solutions in the OR creates a unique situation in which the perioperative nurse must ensure the utmost safety for the patient. Once a medication or solution is removed from its original container, the identity of that product is lost. Some medications are clear and there is no way to discern one medication or solution from another without some form of identification. Errors have occurred because of improper labeling, lack of labeling, or poor labeling of medications and solutions used on the sterile field. The ultimate tragedy has been death because of poor practice. Labeling properly is a risk reduction strategy that is the responsibility of all surgical team members. Using customized preprinted labels may be one method that can help promote compliance with this standard.

As described earlier, JCAHO provides and updates National Patient Safety Goals annually. The 2007 goal specific to medication and solution labeling is goal #3: Improve the Safety of Using Medications, Requirement 3D: "Label all medications, medication containers (for example, syringes, medicine cups, basins), or other solutions on and off the sterile field." (JCHAO, 2006).

The implementation expectations for this goal are very clear. These guidelines should be followed when using medications and solutions on and off a sterile field:

- Label all medications and solutions both on and off the sterile field, even if there is only one medication being used.
- Label when a medication or solution is transferred from the original packaging to another container.
  - Include on the label the drug name, strength, amount (if not apparent from the container), expiration date if the drug is not used within 24 hours, and expiration time if the expiration occurs in less than 24 hours.
- Verify labels both verbally and visually with two qualified individuals when the person preparing the medication is not the person administering the medication.
- Label each medication as it is transferred to another container and label only one medication at a time.
- Discard any unlabeled medications or solutions immediately.
- Keep the original medication/solution container in the procedure room until the end of the procedure.
- Discard or remove all labeled containers from the sterile field at the conclusion of the procedure.
- All medications and solutions on and off the sterile field should be reviewed by exiting and entering personnel during any change in personnel, such as at shift change or break relief.

The perioperative nurse has a significant role in promoting medication safety. Review of the AORN Guidance Statement, Safe Medication Practices in the Perioperative Settings Across the Life Span (AORN, 2006) will provide valuable information to educate the perioperative nurse on this very important aspect of patient safety.

Document Intraoperative Activities: Document Solutions Used and Medications Administered

Documentation of all medications administered during the surgical procedure is necessary to ensure continuity of care throughout the patient's perioperative experience. Should a medication-related event occur at any time during the perioperative period, this information becomes critical. Timing of medications related to a dosing schedule will be based on prior documented doses. Careful documentation should include the name of the medication or irrigating solution, dose, and route of administration.

Perform Counts

Principles of Patient Safety

A retained foreign body can result in significant injury. The primary purpose for performing counts is to avoid this situation and provide for the patient's safety throughout the intraoperative phase (AORN, 2006). Sponge, sharps, and instrument counts are performed for all procedures in which these items could be retained in a body cavity.

There are general guidelines that the perioperative nurse should consider when performing counts for all three of these categories.

- The scrub and circulator should count in unison and aloud while the scrub touches each item.
- Do not interrupt the counting procedure.
- If either party is unsure about a count, the count should be performed again.
- The circulating nurse should record the results of the count immediately.
- The circulating nurse should add to the original count when additional sponges, sharps, or instruments are dispensed during the surgical procedure.
- The names of the scrub person and the circulating nurse should be recorded as soon as each count is completed.
- When a change of personnel occurs, counts should be performed.
- After the initial count is performed, no trash or linen should be removed from the surgical suite until the patient leaves the room (Rothrock & Smith, 2003).

Policies should be in place for performing counts and for actions to take when a discrepancy occurs.

The perioperative nurse takes responsibility to ensure that the proper counts are taken before the surgery begins and at closing of the surgical site. A worksheet is usually used to document the initial sponge and sharps count, separating out the type of sponges and numbers and types of sharps (e.g., suture needles, hypodermic needles, scalpel blades). An instrument inventory/count sheet is often available with each instrument set for counting instruments.

Document Intraoperative Activities: Document Counts

Evidence that counts were correct at the conclusion of surgery must be present in the patient's medical record. Documentation of the final count includes the date (this may be on the record somewhere other than the count area); type of count (sponge, sharps, instrument); count correct or discrepancy; names of those involved in the counting procedure; and if a discrepancy occurs, what action was taken.

Example:

5/4/06 Sponge and sharps count correct. J. Doe, RN, CNOR/M. Smith, CST

7/2/06 Sponge count correct. Sharps count discrepancy. Surgeon notified. X-ray taken, no sharps detected. I. Jones, RN, CNOR/J. Doe, RN, CNOR

Perform Universal Protocol (e.g., Time Out)

Universal protocol is implemented to ensure patient safety. Specifically, adherence to the protocol's requirements is an important and necessary tool in the prevention of wrong site, wrong patient, and wrong procedure surgery. As the primary patient advocate, the perioperative nurse is responsible for ensuring strict compliance with facility policies and procedures that detail implementation of the universal protocol.

Legal Responsibilities and Implications for Patient Care

On July 1st, 2004, the Joint Commission on Accreditation of Healthcare Organizations (JCAHO) mandated adherence to the universal protocol as a necessary requirement for accreditation. In response to this directive, all health care facilities developed methodology and procedures to implement the protocol. The protocol was developed with expert input from various relevant clinical specialties and disciplines, and is endorsed by numerous medical associations (JCAHO, 2006). Development of the protocol focused on reaching a consensus as to what issues were mutually regarded as most relevant to improving patient safety and preventing wrong site surgery events. Participants then developed specific steps based on the principles identified as most important. From these initial recommendations, a universal protocol evolved. The current protocol includes the following requirements (JCAHO, 2006):

- **A defined preoperative verification process must be in place.** The process must ensure availability of tests and relevant studies for review. Data should be reviewed before the start of the procedure for consistency with the planned surgical procedure. Discrepancies or questions regarding site, procedure, or the availability of requested equipment or implants should be addressed before proceeding with the intervention.

- **The operative site should be marked before the procedure** for all interventions involving laterality (right/left), level (spine), or multiple structures (fingers, toes). The mark should identify the site or sites of incision. Marking should be done by the person who will be performing the procedure, involve the patient when possible, and take place in a location outside the room where the procedure is to be performed. The mark should remain visible after the surgical prep is completed.

- **A time-out procedure should be performed before the surgical incision is made,** and should include active participation of all surgical team members.

Specific data elements required for the time-out are delineated in the following section.

Diagnostic Procedures and Results; Surgical Procedure; Expected Outcomes Related to Identified Interventions

The professional perioperative nurse implements recommended practices and follows institutional procedures designed to protect the surgical patient from injury related to wrong site, wrong procedure occurrences. The nurse identifies the patient using verbal and visual verification of unique patient identifiers. Appropriate identifiers are dictated by institutional policy and may include identification band, birth date, medical record number, and family and patient verbalization of identity. The perioperative RN employs active listening skills to gain information regarding the patient's understanding of the scheduled procedure. The patient's medical record is reviewed for diagnostic test results, physician notes, history and physical, and surgical consent forms.

The surgery schedule is checked for agreement with the surgical consent, and the nurse verifies the availability of any requested implants or equipment. All information is reviewed and assessed for relevance and agreement with the proposed surgical intervention. Any discrepancy or disagreement noted after the medical record review, or the patient's verbalization as to understanding of the procedure, is cause for delay of the procedure. The surgeon is consulted and the discrepancy is either resolved or results in cancellation of the scheduled surgery.

Specifics of site marking are delineated in the preceding paragraphs. Facility policies describe protocols for marking of patients. The perioperative nurse demonstrates knowledge of procedural issues and ensures compliance with institutional safeguards regarding marking of the surgical site.

Time-out procedures are performed before the surgical incision and involve active communication with all members of the surgical team. The RN initiates the time-out and verifies the consensual agreement of the surgical team as to the planned surgical procedure. JCAHO requirements define specific data elements that must be included in the time-out procedure:

- identification of patient,
- operative side/site,
- surgical procedure,
- patient position, and
- availability of specific implants or equipment.

All health care organizations should have policies in place to define actions to be taken in the event of a discrepancy or lack of agreement during the time-out procedure (JCAHO, 2006). Protecting the patient from harm related to wrong site surgery demonstrates the perioperative nurse's ability to maintain the safety of the intraoperative environment. An applicable PNDS outcome statement/ definition might be "the patient is free from signs and symptoms of injury due to extraneous objects, e.g., instruments, equipment, or sharps" (Kleinbeck, 2005).

Document Intraoperative Activities: Document Universal Protocol

Regulatory Standards and Voluntary Guidelines (e.g., AORN Standards, Recommended Practices and Guidelines; JCAHO)

To ensure compliance with JCAHO requirements, all events related to performance of the time-out procedure must be documented according to facility policies governing documentation. Many institutions use a preprocedure checklist, while others have developed combination preoperative checklist/time-out verification forms. Regardless of the format, certain data elements must be verified and recorded. These elements include, but are not limited to, the following:

Preoperative data elements:

- Verification of patient identity
- Verification of informed surgical consent/agreement as to scheduled procedure verified with patient or designee
- Verification of surgical site/side
- Verification of review of history and physical, applicable diagnostic tests, physician orders/comments
- Verification of availability of necessary implants or equipment

Intraoperative data elements:

- Verification of patient identity
- Verification of informed surgical consent/agreement as to scheduled procedure verified with surgical team
- Verification of surgical site/side
- Verification of patient position
- Verification of availability of necessary implants or equipment

The perioperative registered nurse follows recommended practices for documentation and maintenance of an environment conducive to optimal patient safety outcomes.

Document Intraoperative Activities: Maintain Accurate Patient Records

Reporting Techniques to Multidisciplinary Health Care Providers (e.g., critical lab values; medical condition; medications; allergies; implants/implantable devices; hand off; read back verbal orders; communication barriers)

Communication of issues affecting the surgical patient directly affects the quality of the patient's outcomes. Medical errors are responsible for thousands of patient injuries each year. Many of these mistakes occur due to sloppy or inaccurately documented patient data. Inaccurate documentation involves errors of omission and commission. Maintenance of accurate data requires careful attention to detail. The perioperative professional has an obligation to document and maintain an accurate record of all data affecting the care of the surgical patient.

An isolation patient arriving in a crowded recovery room, with no documentation as to the need for isolation procedures, can profoundly affect the delivery of care for every patient and employee who becomes unwittingly exposed. The nurse who forgets to detail a skin tear over the coccyx that occurred during positioning of the patient may be responsible for any further skin breakdown that occurs while the tear goes unnoticed. Failure to accurately document blood loss may result in a patient who suffers from complications related to hypovolemia.

Accurate documentation of patient data is important both to the prevention of medical errors and to the timely treatment of patient complications. Patients with multiple allergies that may include latex, antibiotics, and narcotics are a challenge to health care providers. Careful verification of all allergies is vital to the safe care of such patients. Patients arriving in the intraoperative environment with implantable devices such as an automatic implantable cardiac defibrillator (AICD) require special attention. Failure to properly document and communicate the presence of this device to the next caregiver could have disastrous results for the patient.

The perioperative nurse functions in multiple roles throughout the surgical intervention. While accuracy of documentation is important throughout the health care setting, the perioperative environment challenges the nurse to prioritize actions and use effective organizational and time-management skills to maintain the accuracy and completeness of the patient record. Some common intraoperative data elements requiring particular attention to accuracy, detail, and communication include:

- blood loss,
- presence of implantable devices,
- allergies,
- isolation precautions,
- adverse reactions to medications,
- injuries to skin integrity,
- nonsurgical fractures or joint limitations,
- language barriers and other sensory impairments, and
- mental status.

Instruments, Supplies, and Equipment Relating to Surgical Procedure; Implants (e.g., handling; tracking; sterilization)

Accurate recording of use of patient supplies and related equipment is important to proper billing and reordering functions. Facility policies define methods for intraoperative recording of implantable devices and prostheses, and Chapter 6 addresses recommended practices and data elements specific to the sterilization, handling, and tracking of implants. The perioperative RN practices patient advocacy by maintaining an accurate record of all relevant patient data. In this way, the patient is protected from harm due to future adverse events related to improper billing, sterilization issues, or implant recalls.

Document Intraoperative Activities: Document All Relevant Facts and Data Elements

Documentation of All Nursing Interventions

Intraoperatively, the perioperative nurse performs ongoing assessments and intervenes to adjust the plan of care through analysis of patient responses. Documentation is a vital link in the communication and evaluation of surgical interventions. The nurse is responsible for recording all interventions, responses, adverse occurrences, and any other pertinent data elements. In addition, the names of all personnel participating in the procedure must be noted on the patient record. The importance of documentation to optimal care of the patient cannot be overstated. After the surgical patient is transferred to the postoperative area, the operative record is accessed as a reference tool to assist in delivery of appropriate care. Missing or incomplete data can affect the course of the patient's recovery and outcome.

The operative record also stands as a legal document detailing perioperative events. The old adage "if it wasn't documented, it wasn't done" is very applicable in both the health care and courtroom setting. Part of patient advocacy consists of completing the patient record in a manner that thoroughly describes all components of the surgical event. Detailing the numerous measures implemented intraoperatively to protect the surgical patient from harm is an important obligation of the professional perioperative nurse.

Methods of recording documentation vary by institution. Many hospitals are moving to electronic/computer-based systems for documentation of patient care. Regardless of the manner of recording, all intraoperative records should contain a patient-specific care plan that reflects appropriate perioperative diagnoses, risks, interventions, and outcomes. The care plan must be personalized for the individual patient and allow for recording of all pertinent data. A partial list of some relevant data elements routinely recorded follows.

- Performance of universal protocol (e.g., time-out procedure)
- Skin preparation solution
- Surgical position and positioning devices
- Tourniquet application/times of inflation and deflation
- Safety devices (e.g., grounding pads, bed straps, anti-embolism stockings)
- Preoperative and postoperative skin condition
- Sponge, sharps, and instrument counts
- Wound class
- ASA status
- Surgery times (e.g., in room, incision, closure, out of room)
- Equipment identification numbers (e.g., power units, electrosurgery devices, tourniquets, warming devices)
- Intraoperative medications
- Administration of blood products; blood loss/urinary output
- Fluid totals and types (IV and irrigation)
- Preoperative and postoperative diagnosis
- Surgical procedure performed/complications
- Implants of any type
- Existing physical or sensory impairments (e.g., hard of hearing, limited range of motion, language barrier)

Performing and Documenting Sterilization Procedures

The perioperative nurse records and documents evidence of sterilization according to facility policies and procedures. Recording sterilization data offers verification of maintenance of the sterile field. In addition, it permits evaluation and analysis of the process in the event of an adverse postoperative event such as surgical site infection. Chapter 6 discusses specifics of methods of sterilization and the required processes, times, and indicators.

Document Intraoperative Activities: Record Unusual Occurrences and/or Variances in Care

Legal Responsibilities and Implications for Patient Care; Documentation of All Nursing Interventions

Throughout the perioperative experience, opportunities exist for untoward effects or unusual occurrences to occur. These are often referred to as variances or occurrences. The perioperative nurse must be aware of these occurrences or variances from normal and document them appropriately. Documentation of the perioperative phase includes many facets, which are discussed in this chapter. This particular section discusses unusual situations that must be documented and how to document them.

When an unusual event occurs, details must be entered in the operative record completely, accurately, and in a factual manner (Rothrock & Smith, 2003). The writer should not include interpretation, judgment, or opinion. A variance should be reported to the unit director immediately and actions taken to remove defective equipment or supplies until further investigation is completed.

The occurrence may or may not result in patient injury. Regardless of the outcome, a variance report should be completed. Most hospitals have a pre-printed form that is used to document the details of the occurrence. This form is then kept by the risk management department for use in review of incidents and for any legal proceedings that may result. The nurse should never document in the patient's medical record that a variance report was completed. Several situations in which a variance report is written include:

- falls;
- injury to a patient;
- needle sticks or sharps injury;
- fire;
- malfunctioning equipment;
- medication error;
- medication reaction;
- lost sponge, needle, or instrument during a procedure (unresolved count); and
- retained item in a patient.

There may be other situations in which a variance report is completed. The perioperative nurse must be aware of any situations that may result in unfavorable or unexpected outcomes and document such on the report.

Documentation can sometimes be stressful when trying to avoid subjective points or judgments related to the situation. The following are examples of appropriate documentation.

Example 1:

Documentation on patient record:
- "Grounding pad removed at end of procedure. Reddened, mottled area noted under pad area approximately 2 inches by 3 inches at the distal end of the pad site. Dr. Smith notified."

The variance report contains details that are more specific:

- "Grounding pad removed at end of procedure. Reddened, mottled area noted under pad area approximately 2 inches by 3 inches at the distal end of the pad site. Dr. Smith notified."
- "Electrosurgery unit #5 removed from service and sent to biomedical department for evaluation. Grounding pad serial number 453S2. All other grounding pads with same serial number quarantined."

Example 2:

Documentation on patient record:

- "Patient turned onto recovery bed from prone position at end of procedure. Reddened area noted on left knee, anterior aspect, approximately 2 inches in diameter. Dr. Jones notified and examined area."

Variance report documentation:

- "Patient turned onto recovery bed from prone position at end of procedure. Reddened area noted on left knee, anterior aspect, approximately 2 inches in diameter. Dr. Jones notified and examined area. Positioned for surgery using gel pads on both knees. Positioning checked by Dr. Jones prior to beginning procedure. Gel pads intact and remained on knees throughout procedure with no evidence of breaking or leaking. Gel pads removed for further inspection. No other reddened areas noted."

The variance report gives as much detail as possible about the situation, preparation for the procedure, and follow through after the occurrence. The purpose of the variance is to provide details weeks, months, or years after the actual occurrence; therefore, it is imperative that the perioperative nurse take responsibility for clear, concise, accurate, and factual documentation.

Document Intraoperative Activities: Document Maintenance of a Safe Environment

Expected Outcomes Related to Identified Interventions; Physiology Responses to the Surgical Experience Including Potential Complications; Principles of Positioning

The *Perioperative Nursing Data Set* (PNDS) can be used to provide guidelines for complete, accurate documentation of the intraoperative phase of care. Included in this documentation are the aspects of care that ensure and maintain a safe environment. Documentation must be thorough, factual, and complete. This is achieved by addressing the nursing diagnoses, interventions, and both desired and actual outcomes. The PNDS attaches a code to the diagnosis (X), nursing interventions (I), and outcomes (O) (Beyea, 2002).

Specific PNDS nursing diagnoses that should be used in the intraoperative documentation related to safety include:

- Risk for injury related to transfer and transport (X29);
- Risk for infection related to invasive procedures (X28);
- Risk for impaired skin integrity related to immobilization, pressure, and/or shearing forces (X50); and
- Risk for injury related to surgical environment, extraneous objects, and equipment (X29).

The nursing interventions related to each of these nursing diagnoses are too numerous to list here, but they include all of the activities of the perioperative nurse discussed in this chapter. Items included in "documentation of activities to maintain safety" include use of safety devices, such as safety straps; protective measures when using the laser, electrosurgery, and tourniquets; methods for moving and positioning the patient; and counts performed and correct.

Examples of documentation related to specific PNDS intervention statements are:

- "Implements protective measures to prevent injury due to electrical sources" (I72) includes such items as the electrosurgery unit number; the cut/coagulation settings; mode (bipolar, monopolar); the pad lot number, pad site and appearance before and after use, and who applied the pad.

- "Performs required counts" (I93) documentation includes count correct, yes or no; surgeon notified of counts; actions taken for unresolved counts; and names and titles of personnel performing the count.

Document Intraoperative Activities: Document Patient Outcomes

Expected Outcomes Related to Identified Interventions; Physiology Responses to the Surgical Experience Including Potential Complications; Postoperative Complications

The intraoperative care plan reflects an assessment by the perioperative nurse and details nursing diagnoses and interventions designed to protect the patient. The impact and effectiveness of the designed interventions are described as outcomes. The nurse plans care to achieve a desired, or expected, outcome. The nurse functioning in the intraoperative environment continually monitors the responses of the surgical patient. Operative nursing care is focused on adapting to the unique physiologic and psychological responses of the individual patient. Physiologic responses to surgical intervention vary greatly, and while somewhat predictable, reflect individual and idiosyncratic differences. The perioperative professional adapts and adjusts interventions to provide safety and achieve desired patient outcomes. Some instances requiring adjustment of planned interventions might include:

- allergic or toxic reaction to pharmacologic agent;
- sponge or instrument count discrepancy;
- intraoperative hemorrhage;
- damage to skin integrity during transfer or positioning;
- loss or obstruction of airway;
- break in aseptic technique;
- intraoperative cardiac arrest;
- malignant hyperthermia (MH) crisis;
- positioning difficulties secondary to impaired physical mobility; and
- intraoperative findings that alter planned surgery (e.g., undetected metastasis, tumor, abscess, abnormality).

All intraoperative care plans should detail outcomes and allow for documentation of individual patient responses. The nurse has an obligation to accurately describe the effects of interventions applied during the surgical event. Careful documentation of intraoperative responses and occurrences are important to the expectation of postoperative outcomes (e.g., the patient who suffers a skin tear will require attention to the injury site; the patient with an aseptic technique break will require adjusted antibiotic prophylaxis; the patient with temporary loss of airway will require neurologic and respiratory evaluation).

Resources for Professional Growth; Nursing Research and Evidence-Based Practice

The PNDS vocabulary describes surgical patient outcomes related to perioperative-specific nursing diagnoses and interventions. Use of the PNDS supports a consistent description of the comprehensive series of events occurring throughout the perioperative patient journey. For instance, use of the word "signs" in an outcome statement refers to observable or objective effects, while the word "symptoms" suggests more subjective, patient-described phenomena (Kleinbeck, 2005).

Patient care is focused on four domains, or areas of intraoperative concern, which include safety, physiologic response, behavioral response, and health system. Surgical care plans using this standardized terminology promote the acceptance of the PNDS as the universal language of perioperative nursing. Examples of PNDS vocabulary describing patient outcomes might include the following:

- "the patient is free from observable signs of injury related to use of electrical devices"—Safety domain
- "the patient is free from numbness or pain associated with use of positioning devices"—Safety domain
- "the patient's wound is closed and covered with a sterile dressing upon transfer to PACU"—Physiologic responses domain
- "the patient remains unable to move lower extremities secondary to spinal anesthesia upon discharge from OR"—Physiologic responses domain
- "the patient verbalizes understanding of realistic expectations for post-surgical recovery"—Behavioral responses domain (Kleinbeck, 2005).

Document Intraoperative Activities: Document Surgical Wound Classification

Quality Improvement Principles; Expected Outcomes Related to Identified Interventions

Surgical wound classification is an important tool in the evaluation of risk for postoperative infection. Accurate identification of wound class is crucial to the validity of patient outcome studies. Educational efforts directed at clinical professionals responsible for identifying and classifying surgical wounds should be ongoing, based on current research and recommended practices. Establishing a method to review accuracy and allow feedback from both staff members and reviewers is one way perioperative educators can increase awareness as to the importance of proper wound classification.

Classification of a surgical wound is an attempt to determine the bacterial load (i.e., level of contamination) present in the surgical wound. Wounds have been classified by level of risk for contamination since a 1964 National Academy of Science study (Devaney & Rowell, 2004). Over the years, other studies have looked at associated issues such as length of surgery and anesthesia and antibiotic choice and timing as contributing factors in estimating the potential risk for wound infection. Including these factors along with some measure of patient/host resistance spawned research demonstrating that measurement of multiple variables such as these provided a better predictive tool for wound infection than measurement of wound class alone (Devaney & Rowell, 2004). Wound classification data is an important component of current research projects and studies related to patient outcomes.

Multidisciplinary Services (e.g., wound care); Implications for Patient Care

Proper identification of wound class is a required competency for the perioperative professional. In the intraoperative phase, the RN recognizes that properly classifying the surgical wound requires ongoing assessment and input form the surgical team. A wound that appears to fall under the Class 2 (Clean/Contaminated) category can quickly become a Class 4 (Dirty/Contaminated) case with the discovery of an abscess or pus in the surgical wound. The perioperative nurse engages the cooperation of the surgical team in the effort to accurately document the wound class.

Most hospitals use a standardized system for documenting wound class. The CDC offers a guideline to describe surgical wounds. This tool defines four wound categories. A summary of these classes, differential features, and some common procedures associated with each, is found below (CDC, 2006):

Class 1—Clean
- Description: Uninfected wound; no inflammation; no entry into respiratory, gastrointestinal or genitourinary tracts; wounds are closed primarily
- Common procedures: Routine laparotomy; breast or neck dissection; nonpenetrating blunt trauma; total joint replacements

Class 2—Clean/Contaminated
- Description: Involves entry into respiratory, gastrointestinal or genitourinary tract; no evidence of unusual contamination, break in technique or infection is noted; may commonly involve: appendix, vagina, oropharynx, biliary tract
- Common procedures: Cholecystectomy (all approaches); panendoscopy; routine appendectomy or small bowel resection; cystoscopy

Class 3—Contaminated
- Description: Open, fresh, accidental wound (open fractures); major breaks in technique spillage from gastrointestinal tract; acute, non-purulent inflammation
- Common procedures: Reduction of open fractures; appendectomy for inflamed appendicitis; laparoscopic cholecystectomy with bile spillage

Class 4—Dirty/Infected
- Description: Wounds with retained, devitalized tissue; existing clinical infection; perforated viscera
- Common procedures: Incision and drainage of abscess; perforated intestine; peritonitis; debridement of decubitus ulcer; tonsillectomy for chronic, infected tonsils

The perioperative RN uses knowledge of institutional policies and follows approved procedures for documenting wound class. The nurse recognizes that postoperative protocols related to antibiotic use or dressing changes may be predicated on the degree of wound contamination. As the primary patient advocate, the RN demonstrates critical thinking and incorporates intraoperative findings in the assessment and documentation of proper wound classification.

Examples of cases and proper wound class documentation:

"Routine laparoscopic cholecystectomy" = wound class 2
Why? Procedure involves entry into gastrointestinal tract.

"Tonsillectomy" with a preoperative diagnosis of "chronic, infected tonsils" = wound class 4
Why? Procedure involves presence of existing clinical infection.

"Open reduction, internal fixation, compound ankle fracture" = wound class 3
Why? Fracture is open and accidental.

Document Intraoperative Activities: Document Implanted or Explanted Devices

Implants, Regulatory Standards and Voluntary Guidelines, Requirements of Handling Specimens, Reporting Techniques to Multidisciplinary Health Care Providers

A variety of items may be surgically implanted in a patient for various reasons. Some examples of implants include plates and screws for fracture fixation; total joint prostheses; electronic devices such as a defibrillator, vagus nerve stimulator, or spinal cord stimulator; bone; tissue, such as a cornea or patellar tendon; vascular grafts; ports for vascular access; and pain pumps.

The perioperative nurse must ensure that any item implanted into a patient is documented on the intraoperative medical record. The documentation should include the item name or description, lot or serial number, size, manufacturer, and expiration date. Some items may have a sticker available with the product that can be placed directly on the record. Electronic documentation, if used, requires entry of all the elements described above into the medical record. The manufacturer supplies a card with the product that is completed after implantation and returned to the manufacturer. The card contains information about the implant, and the nurse adds the patient's name and specific identifiers so that the implant can be tracked back to the patient in the future if necessary.

The U.S. Food and Drug Administration (FDA) and JCAHO have strict guidelines and regulations related to tracking implanted tissue. The institution must retain records that include receipt, storage, and disposition of the tissue. This information must be maintained for 10 years (JCAHO, 2006). Most hospitals create a log of some type in which the surgical staff can document the implant information, date received, storage, implant date, and information about the recipient. The use of electronic documentation facilitates an implant log, because the information entered during surgery is accessible in report form.

Of equal importance is the documentation of items that

are removed, or explanted, during surgery. The item(s) removed is/are documented with as much detail as possible. Usually specific devices will have a permanent serial or lot number visible somewhere on the device. It is more difficult to obtain detailed information for some orthopedic implants such as plates and screws. After the item is removed, the perioperative nurse should ask the surgeon about the disposition of items that do not need to be returned to the manufacturer. Some hospitals require all items sent to pathology for identification and verification even if they are not tissue. Any explanted tissue must be accounted for in the logbook as described above.

Example of documentation of an explanted item:

> "Titanium 3-hole plate and three cancellous 2.0 mm screws removed from left lateral ankle. Sent to pathology per policy."

Summary

The practice of perioperative nursing in the intraoperative phase requires a highly developed combination of knowledge and skills that is unique to this specialty. This chapter reviewed the key aspects of intraoperative nursing activities as they relate to the myriad of safety, physical, psychological, and sociocultural issues affected by the patient's surgical experience. Commitment to patient advocacy requires that the perioperative registered nurse plan and implement effective nursing interventions to promote optimal outcomes.

Case Studies

The following case studies illustrate the synthesis of knowledge and skills demonstrated by the perioperative registered nurse in the circulating role during the intraoperative phase of surgery.

Case Study 1

Mrs. S is a 48-year-old female scheduled for a laparoscopic assisted vaginal hysterectomy (LAVH) this morning. RP, the CNOR-certified registered nurse, arrives in the OR to find her assignment. She is assigned as the circulator for Mrs. S's surgical procedure. RP reviews the scheduled procedure and looks for any special requests that may be noted on the schedule.

RP's first actions after obtaining her assignment are to go to the OR and review the preference card and pick list for this case. She verifies that all items on the lists are included in the case cart that has been prepared by the central service area. RP notes that there are items listed to "have available, but not open" on the preference card. She ensures that these items are in the room and available. This will allow her to remain in the room while the case is in progress, avoiding unnecessary traffic in and out of the room and allowing her to remain aware of the situation in the room at all times.

RP brings the equipment she will need for the case into the room. This includes the video tower, consisting of a video monitor, camera box, video recorder/printer, light source, and insufflator. She checks the equipment before use to ensure all items are functioning properly and verifies that the stickers indicating routine maintenance by the biomedical department are current. While checking the insufflator, she notices that the carbon dioxide (CO_2) volume is low in the tank. She is aware that there is probably not enough CO_2 available to complete the procedure, so she exchanges the tank for a full one before bringing the patient into the room.

RP assists the scrub person with opening the sterile items onto the field. She then continues to prepare her medications, irrigations, and other items she will need to have ready for surgery. The scrub person returns from the scrub sink and dons a sterile gown and gloves. RP ties the scrub person's gown, checks to see if the scrub needs anything at the moment, and leaves to go check on her patient.

RP greets Mrs. S in the receiving area in the surgery department to begin her nursing assessment. She identifies her patient using two unique identifiers, in this case name and birth date. She verifies the proper procedure and site. RP reviews the medical record for allergies, medications that may be ordered preoperatively, particularly an antibiotic, and reviews the surgical consent for the proper procedure and signature from the patient and surgeon.

The anesthesia care rovider arrives in the receiving area to review the specifics of anesthesia with the patient, and RP returns to her room to speak with the scrub person. RP has noticed that her patient is obese and verifies that the OR bed will support the weight of the patient. She then discusses instrument needs with the scrub person. They determine that they have the instruments needed for the procedure, as noted on the surgeon's preference card, and that they are adequate for the patient's size. A set of instruments is available in the event that the procedure becomes an open procedure and RP calls for long instruments to have available as well, because the patient's large size may require instruments that can reach deeper into the abdominal area. RP and the scrub person count sponges and sharps. Both acknowledge that if they need to use the open instrument set, they will count it when it is opened.

RP brings Mrs. S into the room and assists her onto the OR bed. She provides a warm bath blanket to help maintain normothermia and to comfort the patient. She secures a safety strap across Mrs. S's thighs and assists the anesthesia care provider during induction of anesthesia. Once Mrs. S is anesthetized, RP assists with placing her in the proper position for surgery, using leg holders and padding as required to prevent pressure areas. She then evaluates the patient's body alignment and tissue integrity. Because electrosurgery will be used during the procedure, RP applies a dispersive electrode (grounding pad) to the anterior left thigh. She selects this area because it allows good contact with the grounding pad. She noted earlier that there are no metal implants near this site that could interfere with the electric current dispersion through the grounding pad. RP notes the skin appearance and integrity before placing the grounding pad, and she will evaluate the site upon removal of the pad at the end of the surgery. RP or an assistant to the surgeon may perform the prep. She has the proper prep prepared and ready for use.

The scrubbed surgical team enters the room. RP ties their gowns and observes all for any breaks in aseptic technique, which she does continuously during the surgery. Before the incision is made, RP calls a "time out" with the surgical team. Together they confirm the patient, surgical procedure, surgical site, proper positioning, and availability of needed supplies and equipment. As the procedure begins, RP connects the various items from the table to the appropriate equipment: light cord to light source, being careful not to turn on the light until the cord is connected to the laparoscope to avoid fire; camera cord to the camera box; suction to the suction canister; and insufflation tubing to the insufflator, checking to be sure the CO_2 tank is open so that gas is delivered to the insufflator. After all items are connected and turned on, she assists the surgical team with the equipment as needed (e.g., changing insufflator settings or printing pictures).

RP is aware of the patient's condition and the needs of the surgical and anesthesia team throughout the procedure. She provides needed items and assistance throughout the procedure. She documents all perioperative nursing care according to her facility policy on the OR record. RP receives the specimens from the scrub person and places them in the specimen containers, labeling them appropriately for the testing requested by the surgeon. She completes a laboratory requisition for each specimen.

When closure of the surgical site begins, RP and the scrub person perform the closing counts. These include an initial and final count of sponges and sharps. The open instruments were not used; therefore, these are not part of the final count. She reports to the surgeon that both sponge and sharps counts are correct. After the surgery, RP assists during emergence from anesthesia. She helps with Mrs. S's transfer onto the recovery cart, assessing skin integrity and the surgical dressing during the transfer. RP accompanies the patient to the postanesthesia care unit (PACU), where report is given to the RN receiving the patient.

RP then returns to her room to assist with turnover. She helps gather and remove trash appropriately, using personal protective equipment, removes unnecessary equipment from the room, ensures that all medications from the case are disposed of properly, and verifies that the room is disinfected appropriately before bringing in items for the next case.

Case Study 2

Ms. J is a 70-year-old female scheduled for left total hip arthroplasty. She arrives in the preoperative holding area accompanied by her husband and daughter. AC is the RN circulator assigned to care for her during her surgical procedure. After noting the other team members assigned to the case, she proceeds to the assigned OR to begin gathering supplies and equipment.

The surgeon preference card details use of lateral position using a bean bag positioner, overbed arm support, and stirrup leg holder for the skin prep. Sequential compression sleeves, iodine-based skin prep, and intraoperative blood salvage are additional surgeon requests. AC arranges the bean bag on the OR bed, attaching a suction tubing to facilitate use and gathering extra padding materials and an axillary roll to use during positioning. She brings the blood salvage equipment into the room and attaches the disposable sterile kit and required fluids according to procedure.

AC then helps the scrub person check the pre-pulled case cart for completeness and accuracy and open the sterile table. Together, they verify that the correct supplies and orthopedic instrument sets are opened and the appropriate implants are available. While the scrub person is at the scrub sink, AC obtains the necessary supplies for cementing the prosthesis, including bone cement, mixing bowl, and vacuum pedal. She assists the scrub person with gowning, and identifies and delivers sterile irrigation fluid to the instrument table, observing that the scrub person appropriately labels the irrigation.

Preliminary counts are performed and documented. AC understands that limiting the flow of personnel traffic into and out of the room during the procedure is an important factor in the prevention of wound infection. She prepares for the case in a complete manner designed to minimize the necessity of traveling out of the room to obtain additional supplies. Before leaving to interview the patient, AC retrieves the sequential compression device (SCD) machine, verifies that it is in working order, connects the power supply, and places it under the OR bed for easy access.

After checking the identification band, she greets her

patient by name and further verifies identity using the patient's birth date and unit number. She asks Ms. J to verbalize understanding of her scheduled procedure and crosschecks the surgery schedule, consent, and patient description. AC assesses Ms. J's support system through verbal interaction with the family members present. Physical assessment of the patient reveals the following:

- Hypertension—controlled with medication
- Type 2 diabetes—controlled with diet and oral medication
- Body mass index (BMI)—38
- Hematocrit—36; Hemoglobin—12; Glucose—115
- Allergy to iodine
- H/O reflux disease
- H/O pulmonary embolus (PE)

AC communicates with the anesthesia care provider regarding the patient's history of reflux, PE, and allergy. The certified registered nurse anesthetist initiates the ordered IV antibiotic. Before transporting Ms. J to the OR, AC verifies that the surgeon has marked the surgical site appropriately per policy.

Upon arrival in the room, AC informs the scrub person and surgical assistants of the patient's iodine allergy, and instructs the scrub person to remove the iodine-impregnated sterile drape from the custom drape pack. A plain sterile drape is substituted. The iodine-based prep solution is discarded, and an alternate solution prepared for the prep. Before induction of anesthesia, AC applies knee-high pneumatic compression sleeves to the patient's legs, explaining the purpose and rationale to the patient. She activates the machine and observes and checks the setting and function.

AC assists with the transfer of Ms. J to the OR bed. She remains at the patient's side to offer emotional support and reassurance. Because of Ms. J's history of reflux, the anesthesia care provider instructs AC to apply cricoid pressure during induction. AC maintains the pressure until endotracheal tube placement has been verified by the anesthesia provider.

A Foley catheter is placed for intraoperative monitoring of urine output. AC and the surgical team accomplish lateral positioning of Ms. J, with special attention to anatomic arrangement and padding of bony prominences and areas of pressure. A right axillary roll is placed to alleviate pressure on nerves and minimize possibility of brachial plexus injury. The left leg is placed in a stirrup to facilitate surgical skin preparation. After all positioning is completed, AC evaluates the patient's body alignment and tissue integrity, then places an electrosurgery grounding pad on the patient's right posterior thigh. The assistant completes the prep, and AC assists in removing the leg stirrup without contaminating the operative site.

Time-out surgical site verification is performed before the surgical incision. All team members agree as to site, position, patient, procedure, and presence of necessary implants and equipment. The site mark is visible after the surgical prep and is noted during the time out.

AC connects the suction, electrosurgery, and blood salvage equipment from the field. The SCD machine is set for single leg, as the left sleeve was removed after induction to facilitate the surgical prep and intervention. She documents and records all required information and interventions, including wound class, American Society of Anesthesiologist (ASA) classification, equipment numbers, personnel, skin condition, skin preparation agent, position and positioning aids, results of the counts, specimen disposition, and implants. Throughout the procedure, AC monitors and restricts the flow of personnel traffic into and out of the operating room.

During the surgical intervention, Ms. J experiences significant blood loss and her condition becomes unstable. AC assists the anesthesia care provider with additional IV access and fluid and volume replacement measures. It becomes necessary for her to call for help to deliver implants, sponges, and other supplies to the surgical team. Another RN responds and assists the team. Ms. J's condition gradually stabilizes. At completion of the procedure, the surgeon opts to send Ms. J to the intensive care unit (ICU) for overnight observation. AC assists him in locating the family, and he leaves the OR to speak with them.

AC calls the unit to communicate details of Ms. J's surgical complications and condition and allow the receiving unit to prepare for her care. The surgical assistants and nurse anesthetist accompany Ms. J to the ICU. AC completes her intraoperative documentation record and assists with room cleanup and turnover.

Suggested Learning Activities

- Review the current AORN Perioperative Competency Statements and Recommended Practices.
- Discuss best clinical practices with peers and colleagues.
- Review patient outcome data at your facility in order to identify opportunities for practice improvements.
- Research the literature for evidence-based support of perioperative clinical practices.
- Review facility policies and procedures for intraoperative nursing interventions; recommend updates as needed based on current literature findings.

Chapter 4

Communication

Jim D'Alfonso, RN, MSN, CNOR

Effective communication in the profession and practice of nursing requires a skillful integration of both art and science. Articles and texts abound on a myriad of topics addressing the dynamics and components of effective communication, including basic improvement strategies, conversational styles, conflict resolution skills, delegation, and even the gentle art of persuasion. This chapter addresses effective communication strategies and competencies essential to perioperative nursing practice. These strategies include aspects of effective communication that promote safety, continuity, accountability, and improved patient outcomes for surgical patients.

Novice nurses are typically admonished to heed the age-old mantra, "if it wasn't documented, it didn't happen." Perioperative nurses learn early in their careers that effective communication in the operating room (OR) also mandates an increased awareness of the unique qualities and human aspects of communication, as well as an ability to manage complex relationships interacting in often highly stressful environments. Effective communication in the OR is, therefore, more of an interactive people process than one of documentation.

The rapid pace of change in health care, constant influx of new technology, and complex set of operational challenges that characterize most ORs today must be continually balanced within an environment that is rich with diversity, fraught with distractions, and all too frequently ripe for conflict. Effective communication is in fact a journey and requires a commitment to seek and continually develop a full complement of written, verbal, and nonverbal skill sets that enhance the perioperative nurse's ability to foster an optimal healing environment and safe caring experience that is focused on ensuring quality patient outcomes.

At no time in the history of nursing has effective communication been more closely associated with or directly linked to quality patient care and outcomes. The Joint Commission on Accreditation of Healthcare Organizations (JCAHO) attributes failures or break downs in effective communication for 66% of the nearly 3,000 sentinel events reported between 1995 and 2004 (JCAHO, 2005). These alarming statistics illustrate the importance of effective communication and the need for ongoing competency development to ensure the best possible therapeutic interactions among diverse surgical teams, patients and families, and the health care system as a whole. Many of the National Patient Safety Goals, published annually by JCAHO and available to the public, involve evidence-based approaches to continually challenge, improve upon, and effect change in how surgical and interventional team members communicate vital patient information.

The Association of periOperative Registered Nurses (AORN) supports the integration of National Patient Safety Goals and the expansion of nursing knowledge through the ongoing development of competency, guidance, and position statements, as well as standards and recommended practices. These evidence-based solutions support ongoing competency development in crucial areas such as

- creating a patient safety culture;
- safe medication practices;
- do-not-use abbreviations;
- correct site surgery;
- sponge, sharp, and instrument counts; and
- documentation of perioperative nursing care.

This chapter explores key concepts and best practices and provides a case study that supports the goal of effective communication in surgical settings. Through the consistent integration of these and other best practices, as well as an unyielding commitment to the continuing development of new communication competencies and refinement of related skills, perioperative nurses can continually reinforce patient centered care and create a prevailing culture of safety in the OR.

Learning Objectives

Individuals preparing for the CNOR exam should direct their study activities toward obtaining the knowledge and skills required to communicate effectively in the perioperative environment. Upon completion of this chapter, the individual should be able to:

1. Explore the key concepts of effective communication.

2. Identify best practices in communication that promote

Task/Knowledge/Skill Statements

Communicate patient status and changes to the multidisciplinary health care providers (e.g., critical lab values; medical conditions; medications; allergies; implants)

- Health assessment techniques
- Anatomy and physiology
- Pathophysiology
- Diagnostic procedures and results
- Approved nursing diagnoses (e.g., North American Nursing Diagnosis)
- Transcultural nursing theory (e.g., cultural and ethnic influences; family patterns; spiritually and related practices)
- Behavioral responses to the surgical experience
- Patient rights and responsibilities
- Surgical procedure
- Pharmacology and anesthetic agents
- Pain management
- Preoperative patient preparation activities
- Expected outcomes related to identified interventions
- Physiology responses to the surgical experience including potential complication
- Principles of positioning
- Implants (e.g., handling; tracking; sterilization)
- Communication theories and techniques (e.g., patient/family)
- Interviewing techniques (e.g., patient/family)
- Postoperative complications
- Multidisciplinary services (e.g., nutrition; wound care; social work; visiting nurse; referrals; transportation)
- Surgical consent process

Report

- Health assessment techniques
- Anatomy and physiology
- Pathophysiology
- Diagnostic procedures and results
- Approved nursing diagnoses (e.g., North American Nursing Diagnosis)
- Transcultural nursing theory (e.g., cultural and ethnic influences; family patterns; spiritually and related practices)
- Behavioral responses to the surgical experience
- Surgical procedure
- Pharmacology and anesthetic agents
- Pain management
- Preoperative patient preparation activities
- Expected outcomes related to identified interventions
- Physiology responses to the surgical experience including potential complications
- Principles of positioning
- Implants (e.g., handling; tracking; sterilization)
- Communication theories and techniques (e.g., patient/family)
- Reporting techniques to multidisciplinary health care providers (e.g., critical lab values; medical condition; medications; allergies; implants/implantable devices; hand off; read back verbal orders; communication barriers)
- Postoperative complications
- Multidisciplinary services (e.g., nutrition; wound care; social work; visiting nurse; referrals; transportation)
- Quality improvement principles

→

quality patient care outcomes.

3. Integrate effective communication strategies in contemporary perioperative nursing practice environments.

The Journey of Effective Communication

The ability to communicate thoughts, emotions, and information is a unique characteristic of human beings. Communication, whether verbal, nonverbal, or written, is commonly viewed as a dynamic and lifelong process. The art of communication allows people to convey their basic humanity in the simplest terms, as well as in amazingly eloquent and influential ways.

The foundation for communication progresses with lightening pace from simple sound-bites and fragmented sentences in early childhood to a rich repertoire of complex vocabulary and sophisticated syntax in early adulthood. These building blocks of basic communication facilitate a person's ability to relate or connect with others, as much as it enables them to begin the work of defining "self." The capacity for effective communication continues to expand with both positive and caring interactions, as much as it does with the stressful and more challenging life experiences.

Although life lessons and passive learning may help people make connections and survive, it is through awareness and the conscious pursuit of improved communication that people and relationships truly thrive. An individual's ability to develop and integrate new or different communication skills is not fixed or restricted by age, family patterns, personality type, preferences, culture, habits, or even the ability to speak. When people remain open to and seek mastery of effective communication skills, their prospects

Task/Knowledge/Skill Statements

- Surgical consent process

Document

- Diagnostic procedures and results
- Approved nursing diagnoses (e.g., North American Nursing Diagnosis)
- Transcultural nursing theory (e.g., cultural and ethnic influences; family patterns; spiritually and related practices)
- Behavioral responses to the surgical experience
- Surgical procedure
- Pharmacology and anesthetic agents
- Pain management
- Preoperative patient preparation activities
- Expected outcomes related to identified interventions
- Physiology responses to the surgical experience including potential complications
- Principles of positioning
- Implants (e.g., handling; tracking; sterilization)
- Documentation of all nursing interventions
- Environmental factors (e.g., temperature; humidity; air exchange; noise)
- Reporting techniques to multidisciplinary health care providers (e.g., critical lab values; medical condition; medications; allergies; implants/implantable devices; hand off; read back verbal orders; communication barriers)
- Postoperative complications
- Multidisciplinary services (e.g., nutrition; wound care; social work; visiting nurse; referrals; transportation)
- Quality improvement principles
- Surgical consent process
- Resources for professional growth (e.g., *Perioperative Nursing Data Set* (PNDS); computer skills)
- Nursing research and evidence-based practice

Provide information to the patient and/or family (e.g., status; updates; surgical procedures; reassurance)

- Diagnostic procedures and results
- Transcultural nursing theory (e.g., cultural and ethnic influences; family patterns; spiritually and related practices)
- Patient rights and responsibilities
- Theories of and resources for patient/family education
- Community and instructional resources
- Communication theories and techniques (e.g., patient/family)
- Interviewing techniques (e.g., patient/family)
- Postoperative complications
- Multidisciplinary services (e.g., nutrition; wound care; social work; visiting nurse; referrals; transportation)
- Emergency procedures (e.g., surgical; CPR; MH)
- Regulatory standards and voluntary guidelines (e.g., AORN *Standards, Recommended Practices and Guidelines;* OSHA; JCAHO; ANA Code of Ethics for Nurses with Explications for Perioperative Nurses; state Nurse Practice Act)
- Surgical consent process
- Responsibilities regarding impaired and/or disruptive behavior (e.g., patient/family; multidisciplinary health care team members)

and probability of attaining personal happiness, professional success, and lifelong fulfillment are enhanced.

Although interpersonal communication is a distinctive trait shared only among human beings, there are no innate abilities or birth rights to guarantee that effective communication will one day manifest itself in a person's life. On the contrary—effective communication is a personal journey that requires a conscientious effort, guided by increased awareness, new knowledge, and lots of practice to refine the essential skills that help build bridges and avoid gaps in relating to and understanding others. Nurses must consider all aspects and potential barriers that affect their ability to communicate, remaining aware of the basic components of effective communication, as well as the innumerable barriers that may obstruct or interfere with the process.

Basic Elements of Communication

The basic elements of communication include at least one sender, one receiver, and one message. In perioperative nursing, this process might include a sender (OR nurse) with a specific message he/she chooses to transmit to one or several receivers (a patient, peer, physician, or the surgical team), who upon receipt of the message interprets the message accurately and as intended before translating it into a desired action or response. For communication to be effective, the sender must assume responsibility for the message sent and verify that it was understood by the receiver. This basic process of communication between sender and receiver is intended to

- convey information and
- exchange thoughts or feelings.

The mode or medium by which a message is sent may include verbal, written (paper or electronic), or nonverbal communication (body language). The internal and external climate of communication also exerts considerable influence over the core message being sent, as much as it affects how it might be received. The internal climate is comprised of feelings, values, biases, basic temperament, and stress levels of both the sender and receiver. The temperature, personal space needs, timing, and general surroundings where the communication takes place represent the external environment. There are additional external influences that can lead to potential barriers in effective communication, such as a person's status, power, and authority.

Gender may also come into play, especially when communication and collaboration occur between a predominantly male medical profession and a predominantly female nursing profession. Differences in gender, power, and status continue to affect the overall types and quality of communication from the operating room all the way to the board room.

The actual flow of communication may involve both formal and informal channels, with information traveling upward, downward, horizontal, diagonal, or through the "grapevine." Formal and informal communication networks need to be considered and identified, as they are important parts of mobilizing essential resources and working efficiently within hospital systems that are complex and ever-changing.

Despite the different modes, climates, barriers, and flow that influence the ability to communicate effectively, it is important to remember that communication is first and foremost a human interactive process and that the message being sent is never more important than the people engaged in the process. A hallmark of effective communication is "caring acts in motion," and it requires the nurse to remain vigilant and compassionate in all aspects of relating to others, which in turn helps ensure that the message being sent is the message actually received. Compassion is a key component of all caring interactions, and through intentional application of the knowledge, skills, and attitude required to communicate with confidence and competence, the nurse is prepared to nurture essential therapeutic and supportive relationships that promote the primary goal of effective communication.

Communication Skill Sets

Interpersonal communication skills can be clustered into five key groups that include the following.

- **Listening skills:** Active or conscious skills required to truly understand and effectively respond to what a person is saying.

- **Assertion skills:** Verbal and nonverbal behaviors that allow a person to maintain respect, satisfy needs, and defend rights without dominating, abusing, or controlling others.

- **Conflict resolution skills:** Abilities that allow a person to deal with conflict, while preserving or promoting closer relationships when the conflict is resolved.

- **Collaborative problem-solving skills:** A means of resolving conflict needs and solving problems effectively.

- **Skill selection:** Guidelines that enable a person to choose what communication skills to use in any given situation, including the use of appropriate humor.

Interviewing Techniques

An open-ended interviewing technique is most commonly used. If the patient requires a translator or translation service, the nurse should follow hospital policy and use available resources (e.g., approved translators) and technologies (e.g., two-way language lines) to ensure the patient's individual language needs are appropriately met. Family may provide support for the interview process depending on the patient's age, level of development, or special needs (e.g., child, comatose or disoriented patient), but should not interfere with or respond directly for the patient. There are certain interviewing techniques that can provide valuable insights into a patient's world and help explore their unique and essential nursing care requirements:

- **Silence:** Allowing the patient time to gather thoughts and giving the interviewer time to reflect on what is being said.

- **Facilitation:** Seeking more information or helping a patient elaborate on something said. Facilitation may include a simple nodding of the head or leading statements such as, "I understand," "I see," or "Why is that?" A puzzled look or even a change in position can communicate that the nurse is interested, engaged, and encouraging further dialogue.

- **Confrontation:** Verbal and nonverbal communication can indicate that emotions may be preventing further communication. The nurse must assess the patient's emotional state and may need to confront the patient on possible emotions. Confrontations should be limited to only one topic during an interview to avoid forcing the patient to discuss thoughts or feelings they may not wish to share. Questions such as "You seem anxious" or "You look sad" may promote further discussion and help identify possible interventions to address needs that may have gone undisclosed without gentle and appropriate confrontation.

- **Questions:** Open-ended questioning is preferred over closed-ended questions that require only a simple yes or no response. The interviewer can help elicit more information and promote dialogue by phrasing questions in an open format, such as "Can you tell me what procedure you are having today?" versus "I see you're having a left total knee replacement today?"

- **Direction:** The nurse can help a patient focus on something they stated by asking the patient for further clarification through directing statements, such as "tell me more about that."

- **Suggestion:** Nurses should avoid making suggestions during an interview. Statements like "You have probably had burning in your IV since the nurse added that medication to it?" can promote bias and unduly influence the interview process.

- **Support and reassurance:** In order for patients to share personal and intimate details about themselves, they must first develop some trust in the person to whom they are confiding. Trust can be established through support and reassurance during the interview process. Nurses who demonstrate warmth, honesty, and sincere interest help create a secure environment for dialogue. Appropriate touch may also provide support or restore a patient's confidence, but nurses must be careful not to become overly sympathetic or promise things they cannot control or deliver. Trust and confidence can be lost through statements such as, "Everything will be alright," or "There's nothing to worry about," especially when there may be appropriate reason for the patient to be worried or fearful. Making empty or filler statements can destroy credibility and harm the nurse/patient relationship.

Body Language

Nurses must monitor their own, as well as the patient's nonverbal cues and body language closely. Patients will pick up on subtle nuances and detect incongruent messages, especially when verbal messages don't match visible body language or behaviors. If a nurse gives the appearance of being rushed or distracted, the patient will not believe verbal reassurances such as "I have the time" or "There's no hurry, just take your time" and therefore may not ask questions or make requests to help satisfy their own needs.

When there is an obvious or subtle disconnect between verbal messages and body language, patients will first believe the nurse's body language. Congruent messages should accompany appropriate nonverbal body language. By being aware of the importance of intent and focus, a nurse can help prevent avoidable barriers to effective communication.

Barriers to Effective Communication

The perioperative nurse must remain aware of potential communication barriers that may exist at any point along the continuum of patient care, including those between or among fellow nurses, support staff, other departments, physicians, leadership, or patients. Barriers that challenge the surgical team or serve as communication spoilers might include:

- criticizing—making a negative evaluation of a person;
- name calling—"putting down" or stereotyping;
- diagnosing—analyzing why a person is behaving a certain way;
- ordering—commanding others;
- threatening—controlling by warning of negative consequences;
- moralizing—telling others what they "should" do, preaching;
- praising evaluatively—manipulating through excessive praise;
- excessive/inappropriate questioning—frequent closed-ended questions;
- advising—giving solutions to problems;
- diverting—dismissing problems through distraction or switching topics;
- logical argument—convincing through appeals to fact or logic alone; and
- reassuring—blocking negative feelings or emotions.

Each barrier to effective communication presents its own set of challenges and requires defined skills to help identify, appropriately address, and resolve potential gaps or strife. In assessing patient needs, it is important to identify barriers to communication that could affect a patient's ability to receive and demonstrate understanding of new information. Patient assessment in the perioperative environment should include the following.

- Evaluating a patient's communication skills

- Observing and identifying the patients:
  - age and developmental needs
  - understanding of spoken words and the ability to hear (presence of hearing aid)
  - presence of airway adjuncts (e.g., tracheostomy, laryngectomy, endotracheal tube)
  - presence of alternative methods of speech (e.g., sign language, voice box, keyboard, writing tools)

  - nonverbal clues
  - need for interpreter or alternative direct interpretation (e.g., written literature, telephone service) as needed

- Listening to a patient's speech pattern to identify:
  - age and developmental needs
  - speech patterns
  - clarity of speech
  - complete thoughts
  - grammar and vocabulary patterns
  - discrepancies between words spoken and tone of voice
  - patient comprehension from simple to complex

- Providing for privacy as necessary; allowing patients to share confidential information

- Providing an environment that facilitates understanding:
  - ensures room is quite and has adequate lighting with minimal distractions
  - attracts patient's attention prior to speaking
  - makes eye contact, looking at the patient while speaking
  - speaks clearly and slowly in a moderate tone
  - uses facial expressions, touch, and nonverbal cues appropriately to enhance communication
  - uses visual aids as appropriate to assist with explanations

- Evaluating the patient's response to teaching and interpersonal communication

Conflict or Disruptive Behaviors

Patients and families face innumerable stressors, including fear, anger, and uncertainty over the impending surgery, associated risks, and potential complications. Given these known factors and considering the wide variation of personalities, communication styles, and temperaments of patients, families, and the entire health care team, it is not unreasonable for stress to occasionally reveal itself in disruptive behaviors or outright conflict. In managing conflict, it is important to consider the five basic approaches to handling conflict: avoiding, accommodating, competing, compromising, and collaborating. Given the circumstances and severity of the behaviors or potential for escalating conflict, there may be times when avoiding and accommodating are preferable and appropriate over competing, compromising, and collaborating.

When dealing with a person who is upset or angry, it is best to breathe slowly, speak in a calm manner, and focus on acknowledging feelings (e.g., anger, disappointment, frustration), understanding the situation through listening and providing simple feedback, apologizing without blaming, and explaining what you are going to do to resolve the problem and when you are going to do it. Respecting the person and allowing them to vent or express themselves in a reasonable and appropriate way can help divert anger and conflict into a more positive and constructive exchange. The following guidelines can help work through conflict and seek a true win/win outcome.

- Focus on the issues, not personalities. Avoid saying or doing anything that devalues the other person, makes them feel badly, or places blame.

- Understand the person's feelings by attempting to see things from their perspective. Consider what's important to them and what they have to gain or lose in the conflict.

- Express your ideas and feelings in a positive, constructive manner.

- Be flexible and willing to compromise, by listening with an open mind and a willingness to modify your position based on the other person's input (provided the position is one you feel is fair and equitable).

The goal of effective conflict resolution is to allow a person to deal with conflict, while preserving or promoting closer relationships when the conflict is resolved. The ability to respond effectively to potential anger, frustration, conflict, or other breakdowns in communication can help provide valuable support to the patient, family, and health care team as they return to a more hospitable, safe, and suitable caring/healing environment.

Frameworks for Effective Communication

Nursing has numerous frameworks to support accountability, continuity, and the flow of effective communication between patients, caregivers, and the health care system. Nursing frameworks are the foundation of professional practice and provide a common language, consistent structure, and reproducible process for delivering and evaluating the effectiveness of patient care.

The Nursing Process

The nursing process is included in the conceptual framework of all nursing curricula and is accepted as part of the legal definition of nursing in the nurse practice acts of most states. The American Nurses Association's (ANA) standards of clinical nursing practice incorporate and expand on the foundation elements of the nursing process and include assessment, diagnosis, outcome identification, planning, implementation, and evaluation. These steps provide an efficient, dynamic, and cyclic method of organizing thought processes for clinical decision making and effective communication in nursing. The ANA standards of professional performance include quality of practice, practice evaluation, education, collegiality, collaboration, ethics, research, resource utilization. and leadership. To support these 15 standards, nurses must continually develop and apply effective communication skills in practice (ANA, 2004).

- **Assessment:** The nursing assessment should address physical, psychological, sociocultural, spiritual, cognitive, functional abilities, developmental, economic, and lifestyle aspects. The assessment findings, when combined with medical findings, are then documented in the patient record and form the basis for developing the patient's plan of care. Assessment includes interviewing (subjective data), physical assessment (objective data), diagnostic studies, nursing priorities, and discharge or transfer goals.

- **Diagnosis (problem/need identification):** The process of problem/need identification is a systematic approach to accurately identifying nursing diagnoses. Nursing diagnoses typically change as the patient progresses through various stages of illness; whereas the medical diagnoses may not.
  - The North American Nursing Diagnosis Association International (NANDA-I) clarifies the second step of the nursing process through taxonomy or standardized nursing terminology that helps classify phenomena pertinent to nurses. NANDA-I has approved 167 nursing diagnoses, with definitions, defining characteristics, risk factors, and/or related factors (NANDA-I, 2006).

- **Outcome identification:** A desired patient outcome is the result of nursing interventions and patient responses, desired by both patient and nurse and attainable within a defined period of time, given the present situation and resources. These are the measurable steps toward achieving previously established discharge goals and are important in evaluating the patient's response to nursing interventions. Patient outcomes must: be specific, be realistic, be measurable, indicate a definite time-frame for achievement, and consider the patient's desires and resources.

- **Planning:** The patient's plan of care is based on assessment, diagnosis, and outcome identification. The plan of care is the framework for nursing interventions.

- **Implementation:** This step includes the actual interventions and activities that are prescriptions for specific behaviors expected from the patient and/or actions to be carried out by nurses. The goal of nursing interventions is to provide individualized patient care in order to meet defined patient needs.

- **Evaluation:** Assessment and reassessment provide data for evaluating the patient's progress to a defined clinical standard. If new patient needs or problems are identified on evaluation, then the nursing process would help guide necessary revisions to the plan of care and may include new diagnoses or additional interventions to promote optimum patient outcomes across the continuum of care.

Transcultural Nursing

The use of transcultural nursing theory provides a framework for the development of a culturally competent perioperative nursing plan of care and guides the nurse in establishing mutually defined nursing diagnoses, outcome criteria, and culturally relevant nursing interventions. Culture focused assessment and data collection includes: ethnicity and race, birthplace, communicative competencies, health beliefs and folk practices, religious and spiritual considerations, food preferences/avoidances, socioeconomic considerations, family structure/role, social network, and educational level.

Nursing actions may consist of: encouraging alternative methods of therapy, support for making decisions, delaying treatments until cultural needs are met, permitting cultural healers to enter the perioperative setting to implement health care practices, allowing the patient and family to express feelings, and permitting the patient/family to participate in the planning and implementation of care. Patient outcomes should include expressed satisfaction with treatment modalities and call for open communication between nurse, patient, and family (Rothrock, 1996).

Association of periOperative Registered Nurses

National nursing organizations, such as the Association of periOperative Registered Nurses (AORN), provide guidance statements, professional standards, and recommended practices to support effective communication and the implementation of best practices in a variety of specialties and settings for professional practice. Perioperative nurses should become familiar with and maintain current knowledge of available AORN resources and guidelines as they relate to communication, collaboration, and ethical standards of practice, including:

- competency statements in perioperative nursing,
- guidance statements,
- position statements,

- standards of nursing practice,
- explications for perioperative nursing (with corresponding provisions from the ANA *Code of Ethics for Nurses*), and
- recommended practices for perioperative nursing.

A comprehensive and timely resource to perioperative nurses is the *Standards, Recommended Practices, and Guidelines* manual published by AORN each year. The standards and recommended practices are broad in scope and are attainable, definitive, and relevant to the perioperative setting. They represent an inclusive approach to meeting surgical patients' needs in the practice setting (AORN, 2006).

The Perioperative Nursing Data Set

The *Perioperative Nursing Data Set* (PNDS), developed and published by AORN, is the only nursing data set or structured vocabulary that has the single focus of perioperative nursing and addresses the contributions of professional registered nurses to the care of patients undergoing surgical or invasive procedures. It provides a framework for collecting data that support the importance of professional nurses in the OR and provides a rich data source that helps demonstrate the relationship between nursing practice and patient outcomes. Unlike NANDA, the PNDS incorporates more than nursing diagnoses—its components include perioperative nursing diagnoses, nursing interventions, and patient outcomes. The PNDS is an essential tool for perioperative nursing, with innumerable benefits to clinicians, educators, advanced practice nurses, researchers, managers, and administrators. It provides a standardized method of describing professional nursing care and can be used in communication, documentation, reporting, care planning, or teaching other clinicians and students (Beyea, 2002).

The Forces of Magnetism

The American Nurses Credentialing Center's (ANCC) Magnet Recognition Program offers a hospital or system-wide approach to promote professional practice, recognize excellence, and provide a mechanism for the dissemination of "best practices." Hospitals that voluntarily pursue and achieve Magnet designation through a formal appraisal process must demonstrate a solid foundation and unswerving commitment to quality patient care and nursing excellence, as outlined in the Forces of Magnetism. Key features of Magnet environments include those organizational attributes that reflect open, effective communication in nursing, including high quality patient care, participatory decision making, clinical autonomy, ongoing professional development, two-way communication, collaborative and collegial relationships, and high levels of job satisfaction.

Magnet status is monitored through annual interim reporting, ongoing notification of significant changes in the organization, and a formal redesignation process every four years. The 14 Forces of Magnetism offer a framework to guide an organization's strategic planning in the areas of administration, professional practice, and professional development and support the growth and development of the nursing staff and excellence in nursing services (ANCC, 2005).

Regulatory Agencies

Local, state, and federal agencies outline regulatory standards and uphold specific laws that mandate evidence of effective communication and expectations surrounding the protection of defined patient rights and management of vital patient information. Regulatory standards and legal requirements are typically woven into hospital policies and procedures by designated experts or consultants to the facility who remain current on existing, new, or evolving regulations and laws.

The U. S. Department of Health and Human Services (HHS) is one of the federal agencies that health care organizations rely on for regulatory and legal guidelines. The HHS implements, monitors, and has the authority to levy civil money penalties on entities that violate federal standards and laws, including:

- The Health Insurance Portability and Accountability Act of 1996 (HIPAA);
- The Patient Self-Determination Act of 1990 (PSDA); and
- The Patient's Bill of Rights as defined by the Centers for Medicare and Medicaid Services (CMS).

As licensed professionals, nurses must also remain aware of licensure requirements from state to state. Nurses are responsible for knowing and abiding by licensure requirements and the nurse practice act in the state in which they practice. The over arching goal of regulatory standards and legal requirements is to protect the basic rights of the general public and to uphold the binding covenants between licensed practitioners, health care organizations, and the community at large.

Joint Commission on Accreditation of Healthcare Organizations

The Joint Commission on Accreditation of Healthcare Organizations (JCAHO) maintains standards of quality and patient safety and evaluates an organization's compliance with these standards, as well as other accreditation requirements every three years. The JCAHO standards address an organization's performance in key functional areas, such as patient rights, patient treatment, and infection control.

JCAHO accreditation or certification of special programs can help organize and strengthen patient safety efforts through defined standards and educational resources. The National Patient Safety Goals, Speak-Up Initiatives, Universal Protocol, and the official "Do Not Use" list of abbreviations are a few of the programs and standards outlined by JCAHO. Although JCAHO is a voluntary accreditation process, it is a deeming authority for Medicare certification and recognized by insurers and other third parties that help pay for patient care services.

Community Standards

Community standards may offer additional insight and serve as a source of comparison to standards within a defined health care community or distinct geographical area. Networking through participation in local AORN chapter or state council activities can provide access to valuable resources and potential frameworks used by hospitals or facilities within the community. Neighboring facilities face parallel challenges to implementing new standards, regulations, and policies. Collaboration and partnering among local hospitals can cultivate valuable collegial relationships, expand solutions, streamline implementation processes, and ensure consistency of practice.

Open Dialogue at the Point of Care

Standards of professional practice, regulatory and legal requirements, and hospital policies can help guide the nurse through a myriad of possible interactions, procedures, or processes involved in direct patient care, but they can never substitute for the role of open dialogue in preventing errors or the negative consequences of failed communication. Errors can be avoided only when members of the surgical team work together, communicate openly, and actively talk with each other at the point of care.

Communicating Through Reporting

Reporting may be verbal and/or written with the goal of communicating vital information gathered through the nursing process that is relevant to the patient's perioperative experience and targeted toward optimal outcomes. Informal reporting may be a simple exchange of information between team members with no response or action required, or it may be more formal when patient or process information shared requires a specific and more immediate response or action. Reporting also may include written documentation on designated forms, checklists, or nursing notes that become part of the perioperative patient record. Reports can provide timely information that allows caregivers and members of the interdisciplinary team to respond or act in ways that support patient centered care across the perioperative continuum.

Verbal Reporting and SBAR

Verbal reporting should follow a systematic, organized, and succinct process for sharing information, while attempting to avoid confusion, potential barriers, and break downs in communication. One approach to verbal reporting is SBAR (i.e., Situation - Background - Assessment - Recommendation), which is a rapidly emerging framework for organizing and sharing information between members of the patient care team about a patient's condition. It can be used for framing any conversation, especially critical ones, requiring a clinician's immediate attention or action. It affords an easy way to establish expectations for what will be communicated and how it will be communicated between members of the team, which is essential for developing team work and fostering a culture of patient safety.

SBAR reports to physicians, nurses, or members of the surgical team can be provided in both verbal and written form. Facilities may provide forms to guide the integration of SBAR in planning communication, reporting, and documentation (IHI, 2006). SBAR includes the following basic components.

- **Situation:** Outlines key patient data and specific concerns
- **Background:** Reviews relative findings on the patient's present condition or status and interventions already in place
- **Assessment:** Indicates what the nurse believes to be the problem
- **Recommendation:** Identifies what follow-up actions are suggested

Verbal Orders

Reporting may occur through direct "face-to-face" conversations or by telephone to share information, suggest a particular action, or secure a physician order. Whenever verbal or telephone orders are provided, especially medication orders, mechanisms must be in place to ensure accuracy and safety such as:

- record the order in the patient's record according to facility policy as soon as feasible;
- perform a "read-back" of the written order;
- verbalize the read-back digit-by-digit (e.g., say "one-two," not "twelve"); and
- allow only licensed health care providers to receive verbal orders (AORN, 2006).

Faxed orders or reports should be legible and adhere to hospital policy. If fax orders are unclear, the nurse must request a re-transmission if time permits or revert to a direct telephone order from the physician as outlined.

Reporting involves appropriate communication of findings obtained during initial assessment and chart review, as well as data obtained during ongoing assessment throughout the perioperative process. An important component of assessment is knowing when and what to assess, as well as how and to whom the assessment should be reported.

Reviewing the Patient's Medical Record

A review of the patient's medical record is conducted to ensure that all documentation, preoperative procedures, and orders are completed. Preoperative verification of the correct person using two identifiers (e.g., consent, identification band and patient), the correct procedure, and the correct site should occur in the preoperative area with the patient involved, awake, and aware, if possible. Verification should include relevant documentation (e.g., history and physical, consent), images (e.g., computerized tomography [CT] scans or x-rays) properly labeled, and any required implants and special equipment required for the procedure. The person performing the procedure should mark the site with a "yes" or initials when the procedure involves laterality (left or right), multiple structures (fingers, toes, lesions), or multiple levels (spine). The informed consent and special consent forms (e.g., sterilization consent) are checked to see that they are signed and dated and that they contain witnesses' signatures (AORN, 2006).

Other important elements of the medical record review include the following.

- Identify allergies, including possible idiosyncrasies, and sensitivity to medications, latex, chemical agents, foods, and/or adhesives.
- Identify that height and weight are documented, especially for procedures in which these measurements are important for proper medication dosage calculations.
- Ensure that the results of all laboratory, radiographic, and diagnostic tests are on the medical record. Some of the normal lab values to monitor are listed in Table 1.
- Document any abnormal results and report them to the surgeon and anesthesia care provider.

If the client is an autologous blood donor or has had directed blood donations made, those slips should be present in the chart. Evaluate the most recent set of vital signs and document any significant physical or psychosocial observations. Discrepancies should be reported to the attending physician, anesthesia care provider, and surgical team. Report any special needs, concerns, and instructions (e.g., advanced directives) to the surgical team, including cultural or special needs that might include patients who are Jehovah's Witnesses and do not want blood products, as well as patients who are hard of hearing and do not have a hearing aid with them. Reporting discrepancies or communicating special needs helps the surgical team provide continuity of care while the patient is in the OR (Ignatavicius & Workman, 2006).

Preoperative assessment and reporting should include direct observation, review of the patient health record, and verification with patient/child/family members. Components of the preoperative assessment follow:

- Review the surgery schedule.
- Identify and address barriers to communication (e.g., interpreter services).
- Confirm patient identification:

Table 1
Normal Lab Values

Potassium (K+) level	3.5-5.0 mEq/L
Sodium (Na+)	136-145 mEq/L
Chloride (Cl-)	90-110 mEq/L
Carbon dioxide (CO_2)	23-30 mEq/L
Glucose (fasting)	70-105 mg/dL
Creatinine	0.5-1.2 mg/dL
Blood urea nitrogen (BUN)	10-20 mg/dL
Prothrombin time (pro time, PT)	11-12.5 sec, 85%-100% or 1:1.1 client control
International Normalized Ration (INR)	0.7-1.8
Partial thromboplastin time, activated (aPTT)	30-40 sec
White blood cell (WBC) count/ leukocyte count	Total: 5,000 - 10,000/mm^3 or 7.4 IRU
Hemoglobin, total	Females: 12-16 g/dL Males: 14-18 g/dL
Hematocrit	Females: 35%-45% Males: 42%-52%

  - ensure correct procedure and correct site and
  - encourage patient/family involvement.
- Review the surgical consent form for completeness, accuracy, and congruency with patient's statements.
- Review the preoperative checklist.
- Verify nothing by mouth (NPO) status.
- Verify allergies.
- Review medications taken immediately prior to admission.
- Confirm required diagnostic testing prior to the procedure.
- Ensure that variances from preoperative testing have been reported and addressed.
- Identify cultural, spiritual, or religious needs.
- Confirm preoperative assessment of physical status:
  - weight, height, base-line vital signs, activity level;
  - medical history and physical examination finding.
- Assess physical impairments:
  - hearing, sight, speech, motor ability, neurosensory problems, pain, procedure specific position limitations, drainage, bowel or bladder dysfunction; and
  - verify the presence of prosthetics or corrective devices.
- Assess skin condition:
  - intact, breaks, scars, dry/moist, rash, pale, reddened, bruises, jaundiced, edematous, ulcers.
- Assess mental/emotional status:
  - level of consciousness, responds to name, crying, tremor, anger, talkative, composed, calm, sad.
- Identify iatrogenics (medically ordered devices/measures in use):
  - oxygen, drains, catheters, tracheostomy, nasogastric tube, colostomy, pacemaker or cardiac implanted electronic devices (IED).
- Evaluate patient responses.
- Confirm equipment, implants, and room availability and readiness.

Communication with Family Members

Reporting may include periodic updates to family members in the surgery waiting area. When procedures are scheduled to exceed two hours, it is important to identify (with the patient's consent and participation in the preoperative area as much as possible) when the family might expect an update on the patient's status during surgery and who may be the designated contact person for the family. The designated contact person may provide a cell phone number or pager, especially if they do not anticipate being readily available in the surgery waiting area throughout the duration of the procedure. This information should be recorded in the patient's operative record.

The nurse must remain aware that the family may be anxiously anticipating an update at the mutually agreed upon time. As the designated time approaches, the nurse should communicate that a family update is approaching and clarify with the surgeon and anesthesia care provider what information or status should be shared. When contacting the family in the waiting area, it is important to identify and verify the designated contact person before providing any confidential patient information. Organizational policy should clearly identify appropriate communication strategies to be followed in sharing confidential patient information with designated family or friends by phone, in public waiting areas, and in any phase of the perioperative process.

Relief Reports

Verbal and written reports are an important part of transitioning patient care from one nurse to another, as well as more decisive transitions from one level of patient care to another. Reports are common during the relief of staff in the OR for breaks, lunches, or at the change of shift and are an essential part of continuity of care, safety, and quality. Policies should identify how relief personnel enter and leave the OR during a surgical procedure, such as what counts need to be performed (e.g., sponge and sharp) before relief and the process for reporting and recording counts during the procedure. Relief personnel and the corresponding times they enter and/or leave during a procedure must be accurately recorded in the operative record.

Reports from OR to Recovery Area

The immediate postoperative phase and transition of care from the OR to a designated recovery area may occur while the patient is still emerging from anesthesia, unconscious or unable to communicate effectively. This vital juncture requires open and clear communication with the assigned nurse of the postanesthesia care unit (PACU), intensive care unit (ICU), or other recovery units/sites in the facility where the patient will be transferred. A report may be called prior to the actual transfer (e.g., telephone, intercom, pager) and include projected timeframes for transfer, identification of special equipment, or supply needs (e.g., ventilator, medication pumps, suction, x-ray) and any additional transfer support that may be required.

Report includes the patient's current status, procedure, dressings, intravenous/central lines, drains/catheters, and key preoperative/baseline and intraoperative information that helps ensure continuity and quality patient care during the transition and throughout the postoperative/recovery period. Documentation should support that a verbal report was provided and may include the time, method of reporting, the name and title of the person the report was given to, and any special requests outlined during the report.

The perioperative nurse accompanies the patient to the

designated recovery area and supports the transition through active communication with the receiving nurse and by answering any questions that may arise. When the report is complete and the patient is stable, the transfer is then documented in the operative record and the nurse may then proceed to the surgery waiting area to update the family and provide supportive information on when they may be able to see the patient or how they can contact the recovery area nurse if necessary.

Communicating through Documentation

Documentation of patient care is essential for continuity of care, outcomes determination, quality, and legal protection. Quality documentation should provide:

- better communication of information between the health care team;
- an accurate account of treatment, nursing interventions, and patient responses; and
- disclosure of safety problems, such as change in patient status or risk of injury, early on in the perioperative process.

The documentation of nursing care provided in perioperative practice settings should incorporate the nursing process and be completed for every patient that undergoes surgical or other invasive procedures. The nursing process is the voice of nursing and identifies the critical elements of outcomes-oriented care within a framework that fosters continuity, while allowing for comparison of achieved patient outcomes to expected patient outcomes. Documentation should include information about the status of the patient, nursing diagnoses and interventions, expected patient outcomes, and evaluation of the patient's responses to perioperative nursing care. In using the nursing process, the nurse is able to demonstrate the critical-thinking skills practiced in caring for the surgical patient.

The patient record should reflect a preoperative assessment that addresses physical, psychosocial, cultural, and spiritual needs prior to surgery. The information obtained during the assessment will serve as a baseline for developing the nursing diagnoses and for planning patient care. Assessment is an ongoing process that encompasses the preoperative, intraoperative, and postoperative phases of patient care and actively contributes to continuity of patient care.

The plan of care is based on the assessment and subsequent nursing diagnoses, and it includes interventions that the nurse has identified as actual or potential patient risks/problems. Documentation promotes open communication among members of the surgical team and serves as a legal record of the care provided. Patient outcomes identified by the nurse and included in the plan of care need to be individualized, prioritized, measurable, realistic, and achievable.

Nursing interventions that are performed must be specified in the patient record, including when, where, and by whom during the different phases of the perioperative process. The goals of nursing interventions are to prevent potential patient injury or complications and to intervene or treat actual patient problems. The nurse provides continuous evaluation of perioperative nursing care and the patient's responses to specific interventions. Evaluation is critical to measure the effectiveness of patient care, and documentation offers a means of quantifying actual versus expected outcomes. The perioperative patient record is a valuable tool in conducting performance improvement audits, perioperative nursing research, and risk management.

The perioperative patient record may be recorded on a formal, preprinted paper document or by electronic documentation on a computer. Charting may involve completion by a variety of means, including detailed checklists, narrative notes, diagrams, or "charting by exception." Organizational policy should clearly define the requirements and expectations of documentation and offer guidelines for nurses and members of the health care team in completing the patient's perioperative record.

Perioperative documentation should include, but may not be limited to:

- identification of the persons providing perioperative patient care, such as name, title, and signature of the person responsible for the care;
- description of the patient's skin condition on arrival and discharge from the OR;
- perioperative patient care planning, including baseline data obtained during the preoperative assessment;
- presence and disposition of sensory aids and prosthetic devices, such as eyewear, hearing aids, dentures, or artificial limbs;
- placement of the electrosurgical unit (ESU) dispersive pad and identification of the ESU and settings used;
- use of temperature-regulating devices, including identification of the unit and documentation of the patient's body temperature before and after discharge from the OR;
- placement of the electrocardiogram electrodes, blood pressure cuff, oximetry and temperature probes, as well as any other invasive or monitoring devices;
- patient positioning and/or repositioning devices and supports, including immobilization devices used;
- placement of tourniquet cuffs, including identification of the unit, pressure settings, and inflation/deflation times;

- location of skin prep, including prep solution used;
- use of lasers, including identification of the unit, name of the surgeon and support staff members, type of laser used, surgical procedure, the lens used, length of time the laser was used, and wattage;
- use of intraoperative x-rays and fluoroscopy and protective devices used (if any);
- patient specimens and cultures taken during the surgical procedure;
- location and type of drains, catheters, wound packing, casting material, and dressings used;
- placement and location of implants (e.g., medical devices, synthetic and biologic grafts, tissue, bone) including the name of the manufacturer or distributor, lot and serial numbers, type and size of implant, and expiration date as appropriate and any other information required by the Food and Drug Administration (FDA);
- placement of radioactive implants, including the time, number, location, and type of radioactive material placed in the patient;
- administration of blood or blood products, medications, irrigation solution, and other solutions;
- wound classification;
- anesthesia classification and mode of anesthesia provided (e.g., general, local, spinal);
- documentation of sponge, sharp, and instrument count outcomes as appropriate;
- time of patient discharge, patient status at discharge, patient disposition, and method of transfer;
- any significant or unusual occurrences pertinent to patient outcomes;
- communication with family members or significant others during the surgical procedure; and
- patient and family teaching provided (AORN, 2006).

As an important quality tool, the perioperative patient record may include other elements that require completion by members of the surgical team. The patient record serves as a valuable source for data that support tracking, trending, and evaluation of specific quality or safety measures. The record also should include information on the preoperative verification process, marking the operative site, and "Time out," which comprise JCAHO's Universal Protocol for eliminating wrong site, wrong procedure, and wrong person surgery. The Universal Protocol requires active communication and involvement of the entire surgical team. The "Time out" can be recorded by checklist or other methods specified by organizational policy and must, at the least, include:

- correct patient identity,
- correct side and site,
- agreement on the procedure to be done,
- correct patient position, and
- availability of correct implants and any special equipment or special requirements.

Organizational policies and procedures for perioperative documentation establish authority, responsibility, and accountability and serve as operational guidelines. An introduction and review of perioperative documentation should be included in the orientation process and in continuing education when any modifications are made to the documentation process. Ongoing education provides personnel with the knowledge, skills, and competencies required to document perioperative patient care accurately, completely, and in compliance with defined policies and strategies.

Documentation forms or electronic medical records should include, but not be limited to:

- operative record,
- preoperative patient checklist,
- nurses' notes,
- flow sheets,
- care plans,
- implant records,
- laser logs,
- specimen forms, and
- chain of custody for forensic evidence.

Deaths in the OR

Although deaths in the OR are infrequent and always unsettling, it is important for the perioperative nurse to be familiar with essential documentation that may be required by the health care facility, as well as local law enforcement agencies (e.g., coroner, medical examiner). Organ donation should be considered whenever possible, and collaboration with the appropriate community agencies can help facilitate appropriate evaluation of organ donor options that may need to be reviewed with the immediate family.

Specific forms may be required and should be identified and available in or near the OR suite. Documentation requirements should be outlined in organizational policies that may be seldom employed in the OR, which reinforces the importance of identifying the appropriate policy, seeking support from charge personnel or facility nursing supervisors, and clarifying requirements with all members of the surgical team in managing the death of a patient in the OR.

Communicating with Patients and Families

To promote quality outcomes and meet the needs of patients and their families, communication must focus on creating a climate of trust that includes open communication, establishing rapport, allaying apprehensions, answering questions, active teaching, and providing reassurance throughout all phases of the perioperative experience. The patient is usually concerned about complications, pain, changes in usual activity level, or even payment of the facility bill.

The more extensive the surgical procedure, the more fearful the patient will be in assuming self-care. The perioperative nurse must support the patient and family members as they plan for the procedure and consider discharge needs. The patient with visible scars after surgery may need emotional support from and acceptance of the family. They may be angry about the surgical outcome or about role changes, as well as concerned about financial matters and the ability to return to work. The surgical outcome may not fully meet the patient's expectations, and further interventions may be necessary to assist in resolving these different feelings.

The perioperative nurse must help identify and address these unique and diverse needs as much as possible and often in a very short time frame. It is also important for the perioperative nurse to consider tapping into available internal or external resources that may be able to support the patient and family as needed or more in-depth following surgery (e.g., diabetic teaching, grief counseling, social services).

The teaching plan for the surgical patient and family includes the following:

- prevention of infection,
- care and assessment of the surgical wound,
- diet therapy,
- pain management,
- drug therapy, and
- progressive increase in activity.

It is important to assess both the patient's and family members' current knowledge, as part of the preoperative teaching program. The sequence of events, expectations, and any special care required after surgery can help reinforce teaching that may have occurred before admission and ensure discharge planning is a shared goal between patient, family, and the health care team. Timing and effectiveness of teaching are particularly challenging in outpatient settings, which reinforces the importance of active teaching and discharge planning across all phases of the perioperative process.

Teaching should also include possible signs or symptoms of complications, such as wound infection, and what to do when complications occur. If dressing changes are needed, the patient and family should be instructed in the importance of proper hand washing to prevent infection.

A balanced diet is an important consideration in wound healing; patients should be reminded to follow dietary recommendations and continue supplements, if prescribed, until the wound is completely healed and their physical energy levels are restored. If permitted, patients should be encouraged to drink plenty of fluids and maintain good hydration. Cultural preferences and food practices, as well as socioeconomic influences, also need to be considered.

The patient needs to know about pain medications and the importance of dosage and frequency to prevent "breakthrough" pain. If pain is not controlled or if the pain suddenly increases, the patient should be instructed to notify the surgeon. If antibiotics or other drugs are prescribed on discharge, the perioperative nurse should stress the importance of completing the entire prescription.

Surgery is a major stressor and the body needs time and rest to achieve optimum healing. The patient and family need to know activity levels should increase slowly, rest when tired is crucial, and that all attempts should be made to avoid straining the wound or the surrounding area. The surgeon should identify when the patient may climb stairs, return to work, drive, and resume other usual activities, such as sexual intercourse. The amount of weight a patient can lift after surgery should be specifically defined by the surgeon, and the perioperative nurse can help patients evaluate the possible weight and limits of grocery bags, laundry baskets, luggage, children, and even books. Patients need to consider proper body mechanics, and family members can provide support with adherence to possible restrictions to prevent complications or disability (Ignatavicius & Workman, 2006).

In communicating with patients and families, it is important to encourage questioning and to offer simple explanations free of medical jargon or terms that may be confusing. Documentation of the content shared with patients and families, as well as their response to teaching, is important in identifying statements of understanding direct from the patient, as well as any possible gaps or concerns about compliance. Documentation of teaching and patient response is an important part of accountability and liability for the nurse, particularly with the continuous rise of outpatient surgical procedures each year.

Patients and family also must receive written discharge instructions to follow at home, which may help provide opportunities to review important care information as often as they want or need. Opportunities for demonstration and return demonstration may be feasible for inpatients with ongoing access to professional nursing care, but are somewhat limited for outpatients who are admitted, undergo surgery, and are discharged the same day. Follow-up phone calls and detailed instructions that include contact numbers to call if there are any questions or needs after discharge are an important part of keeping the lines of communication open and supporting continuity, safety, and quality outcomes after the patient returns home.

Summary

Effective communication requires defined skills to send clear and consistent messages to a receiver. Choosing the right communication method and considering other influencing factors (both internal and external) helps ensure the message is received and can be acted upon, if necessary. Through direct application and practice of effective communication skills the perioperative nurse should be able to:

- integrate effective communication processes,
- apply the basic elements of communication in a variety of settings,
- recognize potential barriers,
- send clear and consistent messages,
- use supportive nonverbal cues,
- consider diversity factors,
- actively seek to understand others,
- recognize perceptual influences,
- employ active listening skills, and
- prevent misunderstanding.

Through the continuing development of effective interpersonal communication skills and by choosing the right skill at the right time to optimize results, perioperative nurses can improve their abilities to listen and hear core messages, assert needs without alienating others, resolve conflict in ways that promote shared learning and growth, and collaborate to marshal essential resources.

Poor or ineffective communication skills can result in a wide range of untoward events in the OR, including information or orders that are missed, not conveyed, forgotten, or misdirected. The impact of poor communication can range from simple frustration to a devastating sentinel event. Effective communication is an essential part of safe perioperative patient care, but the potential for errors is ever present throughout the perioperative process and amplified when communication is blocked or absent.

Effective communication helps facilitate patient, family, and interdisciplinary collaboration. The outcomes of effective interdisciplinary communication include improved safety and quality, more effective treatment and interventions, enhanced employee morale, increased patient and family satisfaction, and decreased lengths of stay.

Leadership plays a pivotal role in establishing a culture of effective communication through clear direction, continuing education and role modeling, as well as promoting a deeper appreciation for the many benefits to patient and team. Establishing and maintaining effective communication in the OR is everyone's responsibility, and the likelihood of success increases when people sense they are respected as members of a high performance team with common goals.

Case Study/Discussion Points

A 38-year-old female was admitted to the OR for a scheduled left L3-L4 decompression laminectomy. The consent was confirmed and correct side and level verified verbally and marked with the patient's participation in the preoperative area by the pre-op nurse. X-ray images were with the patient and placed on the viewer in the assigned OR. The OR was set up for a left-sided laminectomy with the ESU and bipolar cautery pedals placed on the floor according to the physician's preference card for a "left" laminectomy procedure. The patient was anesthetized, intubated, placed in the prone position, prepped, and draped by the surgical assistant prior to the surgeon's arrival in the OR.

The surgeon reviewed the x-rays on the viewer and abruptly requested that the nurse move the ESU and bipolar cautery pedals to the other side. The nurse repositioned the pedals accordingly. The surgeon verified the site and side with the anesthesiologist and the surgery began on time. The nurse was out of the room retrieving sutures during the "time out," but documented that the "time-out" had occurred and that all components of the Universal Protocol had been met after verifying directly with the anesthesiologist.

At the conclusion of the procedure, the physician reviewed the postoperative x-rays, history and physical (H&P), and consent forms only to realize he had operated on the wrong side. The patient was taken to recovery, where she was eventually informed of the wrong side surgery, and then returned to the OR for a second procedure.

Discussion Points for Case Study

1. Verifying the correct surgical site at the time of surgery is the responsibility of preoperative registered nurses and every member of the health care team.

2. Active involvement and effective communication are essential to ensure continuity, safety, and quality.

3. Policies and procedures should define who is responsible for marking the surgical site and how the Universal Protocol is implemented. JCAHO recommends that the person performing the procedure should mark the site, which did not happen with this procedure.

4. Multiple checks can help identify if there are any discrepancies between the H&P, surgical consent, patients verbal acknowledgement, and x-ray films. Consistent implementation was not evident in this case and an error in the H&P, performed by a surgical resident, went undetected.

5. Marking of the surgical site and side should be visible after the patient has been prepped and draped. The field was prepped and draped before the surgeon arrived to the OR, and no obvious site or side markings were noted.

6. The surgeon reviewed the appropriate patient films and abruptly requested that the nurse move the ESU and bipolar cautery pedals to the other side, which was in direct conflict to the physician's preference card and long-standing history of where the surgeon preferred the control pedals for a left-sided laminectomy. The nurse thought this was highly unusual and out of the ordinary, but did not raise her concerns with the surgeon who appeared in a hurry and distracted. The pedals were moved, no further questions were raised, and appropriate dialogue did not occur.

7. The nurse left the room briefly to retrieve sutures and when she returned the anesthesiologist confirmed that the "time out" had occurred during her absence. The nurse documented in the operative record that the "time out" took place, although she had not directly witnessed or participated in the process. It is everyone's responsibility to participate in the "time out," and priorities should have prevented the nurse from leaving the room to retrieve suture until after the "time out" was completed. In addition, documentation of the "time out" should have been completed by the anesthesiologist or surgeon who were present and who actively participated in the process. The nurse made a serious documentation error and created an ethical dilemma by completing the "time out" checklist and signing her name, as she unwittingly falsified the patient's operative record

8. Due to the size of the incision and inability of the surgical team to identify the actual side being operated on, the wrong side surgery was not detected until the surgeon completed the procedure and was in recovery reviewing the records and began documenting the postoperative orders. Only at this time, did the team become aware that the surgery had been performed on the wrong side.

9. After a root cause analysis, there were numerous variables that contributed to this wrong side surgery, including failed communication. The policy for wrong site, wrong procedure, and wrong person surgery was carefully revised, education was provided to all members of the surgical team on the importance of active involvement and open communication by all members of the health care team, and regular audits were performed to ensure adherence with the revised policy.

10. As patient advocates, perioperative registered nurses have a duty to protect the patient from injury and to safeguard the patient's health, welfare, and safety. Effective communication, reporting, documentation, and compliance with established standards of practice and hospital policies can support advocacy and ensure patient safety.

Suggested Learning Activities

- Review the current AORN Patient Outcome Standards and Recommended Practices.
- Review your state nurse practice act to know the legal definition and scope of nursing practice.
- Remain aware of the services provided by your facility to improve patient communication (e.g., translators, interpreters).
- Research the literature for information on communication techniques, as well as patient/family interviewing and education strategies.
- Review facility policies and procedures for communication, "time out," and documentation of nursing care—recommend updates as needed based on current literature findings.

Chapter 5

Discharge Planning

Carol Schramm, RN, MSN, CNOR

The responsibility of the perioperative nurse in regard to discharge planning continues to expand with the increase in ambulatory surgery, reduced duration of hospital stays, and the shift of more care to the home environment. Although it may be a primary responsibility of the perianesthesia nurse in many settings, the perioperative nurse also must consider discharge planning for each patient and participate in it. Competency in discharge planning becomes even more important in settings where the perioperative nurse is the only professional nursing contact for the patient. This chapter provides perioperative nurses who are preparing to obtain or renew specialty certification with information about optimal discharge planning.

The Joint Commission on Accreditation of Healthcare Organizations' (JCAHO) *Comprehensive Accreditation Manual for Hospitals* (CAMH) outlines the scope of responsibilities health care organizations have for discharge planning needs of all patients, including those who have undergone operative and invasive procedures (JCAHO, 2006; PC-1). Two core elements identified are providing and coordinating the care, treatment, and services needed by the patient and family. Activities related to those core elements that are associated with discharge planning include teaching patients what they need to know about their care, treatment, and services, as well as coordinating those key elements when the patient is referred, transferred, or discharged. The CAMH further states that these activities may occur over a period of time that ranges from minutes to years, depending on the setting and needs of the patient. Thus, even though the nurse-patient interaction may be brief and focused, there is a clear role for the perioperative nurse to meet the needs of the patient and family and to maintain the continuity of care, treatment, and services.

A wide variety of resources are available to support the perioperative nurse in meeting the discharge planning needs of the patient and family. The nurse must demonstrate competency in knowledge of:

- the nursing process;
- philosophy, definition, and scope of perioperative nursing, as described in the Association of PeriOperative Registered Nurses (AORN) Perioperative Patient Focused Model;
- AORN Competency Statements in Perioperative Nursing, Guidelines for Perioperative Nursing, Standards of Perioperative Clinical Practice, and Outcome Standards for Perioperative Patient Outcomes as described in the AORN *Standards, Recommended Practices, and Guidelines*;
- age-specific and transculturally sensitive learning approaches;
- pertinent state and federal regulatory requirements;
- facility-specific standards of care;
- roles and functions of the multidisciplinary health care team; and
- available community resources.

Perioperative nurses must be able to interpret, synthesize, and apply knowledge from the resources cited above in specific patient situations. This chapter focuses on the necessary knowledge and skills needed by the perioperative nurse for effective discharge planning. Case study situations and specific learning activities are provided.

Learning Objectives

Individuals preparing for the CNOR exam will direct their study activities toward obtaining the knowledge and skills needed for effective discharge planning. Upon completion of this chapter, the individual should be able to:

1. Describe key components of the discharge planning process.

2. Develop an appropriate discharge plan in collaboration with the patient/family and members of the health care team.

3. Correlate achievement of discharge criteria with desired patient outcomes.

4. Assess patient/family readiness to learn.

5. Identify patient/family barriers to learning.

6. Evaluate the patient/family understanding of the discharge plan of care.

Task/Knowledge/Skill Statements

Collaborate with multidisciplinary services (e.g., nutrition, wound care, social work, home nursing care, referrals, transportation)

- Diagnostic procedures and results
- Approved nursing diagnoses
- Behavioral responses to the surgical experience
- Legal responsibilities and implications for patient care
- Surgical procedure
- Pain management
- Principles of patient safety
- Principles of wound healing
- Expected outcomes related to identified interventions
- Documentation of all nursing interventions
- Communication theories and techniques
- Interviewing techniques
- Reporting techniques to multidisciplinary care providers (e.g., critical lab values, medical condition, medications, allergies, implants/implantable devices, hand off, read back verbal orders, communication barriers)
- Postoperative complications
- Multidisciplinary services (e.g., nutrition, wound care, social work, visiting nurse, referrals, transportation)
- Standard and transmission-based precautions
- Quality improvement principles
- Responsibilities regarding impaired and/or disruptive behavior (e.g., patient/family, multidisciplinary health care team members)

7. Identify need for patient referral to other health care team members or services.

A variety of components are central to the discharge planning process. Key aspects of discharge planning include the following:

- assessing the patient and family for postdischarge needs and informing them of options related to diagnoses, prognoses, resources, and preferences;
- coordinating and facilitating the timely implementation of discharge plans and arranging for follow-up care, as necessary;
- maintaining effective communication with other caregivers and family;
- documenting assessment and planning to meet patient and family needs, in accordance with relevant regulatory requirements and facility standards of care;
- providing educational resources to meet patient and family needs and to achieve desired outcomes; and
- participating in multidisciplinary care planning and implementation.

As is the case with most patient care, appropriate discharge planning requires a multidisciplinary approach to best meet all the needs of the patient and family. The Institute for Healthcare Improvement (IHI) is dedicated to promoting patient safety throughout the health care system and has identified that multidisciplinary care planning does not add work to the patient care process, but rather is fundamental to ensuring delivery of the best care possible. However, "today's complex, fragmented systems put great pressure on providers and center care on the needs of the system itself, not the needs of patients" (IHI, 2006). The perioperative nurse must retain the role of patient advocate despite this reality and promote discharge planning that involves all relevant disciplines, whether the focus is on nutrition, wound care, home nursing care, social work, or any other appropriate group of health care professionals.

The perioperative must also be knowledgeable about correlating discharge criteria with desired patient outcomes. Several patient outcomes are especially significant when planning appropriately for discharge, including:

- demonstration of knowledge of expected responses to the operative or invasive procedure;
- demonstration of knowledge of nutritional requirements related to the operative or invasive procedure;
- demonstration of knowledge of medication management;
- participation in the rehabilitation process;
- demonstration of knowledge of wound management; and
- knowledge of pain management.

Effective discharge planning must include having the patient achieve measurable discharge criteria.

Education of the patient and family is central to effective discharge planning and is based on two essential concepts. The nurse must first assess the patient/family in regard to their readiness to learn before moving on to provide education that supports discharge planning. The patient and family may be ready to learn but unable to do so because of barriers to learning, so those impediments must be identified before the teaching plan can be developed and implemented.

Many things can affect readiness or can be a barrier to

learning, so it is crucial to assess the impact of sensory, motor, or mental impairments; ability to speak, read, and write in English or another language; cultural or religious considerations; age-related teaching approaches; comfort measures; and medication regimens, among other things. The nurse must remember that teaching is only complete when the patient and family are able to gain the necessary knowledge and skills needed from the education being conducted.

Discharge planning may address needs of the patient/family as they move among phases of care during an admission, or it may "consist of a clear understanding of how to access services in the future should the need arise." (CAMH, 2006; PC-46). The perioperative nurse must evaluate how well the patient and family understand the discharge plan of care to determine if additional planning or alternative methods must be implemented. If there is inadequate understanding of the discharge plan of care, the patient/family will have no improvement in or may experience a decrease in health status.

The perioperative nurse is but one member of the multidisciplinary health care team that must collectively address the needs of the patient. Depending on the discharge plan of care, there might be a need to involve respiratory therapists, nutritionists, home health care nursing, or a host of other care providers. The perioperative nurse may identify unique needs of the patient related to the operative or invasive procedure, such as implanted devices. Whatever the needs of the patient or family, discharge planning must involve many disciplines to develop and implement the most effective plan possible. Indeed, these needs may extend after the patient has been discharged and far into the postoperative phase during post-discharge follow-up. It is key for the perioperative nurse to receive feedback about the overall discharge planning process to promote more effective discharge planning and to share that with all other disciplines involved.

Collaborate with Multidisciplinary Services (e.g., Nutrition, Wound Care, Social Work, Home Nursing Care, Referrals, Transportation)

Diagnostic Procedures and Results

Diagnostic procedures and results can be key components of the discharge plan of care. The patient may have undergone a biopsy procedure and the results will guide future care, or diagnostic testing may reveal a co-existing problem that had not been identified before the perioperative period. The discharge plan of care must clearly address what is to happen regarding results that are pending at the time of the discharge, such as instructing the patient and family on how to obtain test results or any related follow-up care. It also must include any information regarding care needed for other conditions identified, such as an elevated glucose level and plan for diabetes care.

Legal Responsibilities and Implications for Patient Care

The patient and family are entitled to discharge planning services that are appropriate and individualized to their needs. Federal and state requirements may affect specific components of the discharge plan. The discharge plan must address any aftercare services needed, including the need for supervision after discharge and any support services needed, information about any services that have been arranged, information about medications prescribed and how to use them appropriately, and the plan for any follow-up care that is needed. In addition to rights, patients also have the responsibility to participate as fully as possible in the discharge planning process; the perioperative nurse should encourage this whenever it is feasible.

Approved Nursing Diagnoses, Behavioral Responses to the Surgical Experience

The process of collecting and identifying data in a manner that supports the planning of nursing care is nursing diagnosis. Nursing diagnosis is useful as the perioperative nurse organizes information into actual and potential problems, and then incorporates them into a discharge plan of care. The patient undergoing an operative or invasive procedure will have one or more actual problems, such as urinary incontinence or acute pain—these diagnoses must be addressed by the perioperative nurse. The discharge plan of care also must address the risk for or potential to develop a variety of problems, such as the risk for postoperative infection and the risk for injury related to many perioperative events, such as the use of lasers or tourniquets. In addition, there are many normal and problematic behavioral responses that may need to be addressed in the discharge plan of care, such as anxiety, ineffective coping, and grieving. The nurse may collaborate with other disciplines such as social services or a nutritionist when developing the plan of care. The perioperative nurse can use nursing diagnosis to identify and classify data in a manner that contributes to effective discharge planning for a wide variety of problems.

Surgical Procedure, Pain Management, Postoperative Complications

Appropriate discharge planning for the patient undergoing an operative or invasive procedure must reflect the procedure(s) performed, possible complications associated with the procedure(s), and how to manage any pain that may result. Many facilities develop procedure-specific discharge instructions that include information about what is normal and what is not normal for patients to experience, activity/hygiene restrictions, and pain management. It is crucial for the patient and family to understand what should be happening and what is a complication in order to prevent problems from escalating after discharge. Pain is commonly known as the fifth vital sign, and patients have a right to effective pain management, regardless of how long they remain in the facility after their procedure.

Principles of Patient Safety, Principles of Wound Healing, Standard and Transmission-based Precautions

Patient safety should be a goal for all members of the health care team, and the perioperative nurse can play a major role in promoting it within the framework of the discharge plan of care. The JCAHO focuses on patient safety and publishes National Patient Safety Goals (NPSG) annually. When incorporating patient safety into the discharge plan of care, key considerations include promoting medication safety, reducing the risk of infection, and reconciling medications. The discharge plan of care may involve educating the patient and family about medications for pain and preventing infection. The discharge plan must address educating the patient and family regarding how to take any medications prescribed as a result of undergoing the procedure, as well any potential drug interactions between the patient's routine medications and those newly prescribed. JCAHO's medication reconciliation NPSG is intended to decrease problems associated with multiple medications taken by certain patients. Reducing the risk of postoperative infection is also a NPSG, and the discharge plan of care should include educating the patient and family about the active role they can play in reducing this risk (JCAHO, 2006).

Expected Outcomes Related to Identified Interventions

The discharge plan of care should be based on expected outcomes. Some outcomes may be routinely expected as a result of specific operative or invasive procedures, while other outcomes are individualized to the patient/family. The *Perioperative Nursing Data Set* (PNDS) is a rich source of patient outcomes specific to the perioperative phase of care, including safety/injury prevention, physiologic and behavioral responses, and health system outcomes. The perioperative nurse can use the PNDS to establish general, as well as patient-specific outcomes that apply to all phases of perioperative care, including the discharge planning process. (Beyea, 2002).

Documentation of All Nursing Interventions, Reporting Techniques to Multidisciplinary Care Providers, Multidisciplinary Services

The discharge plan of care should be documented and accessible to caregivers and to the patient and family. Indeed, it is a responsibility incumbent upon health care providers and the facilities that employ them to provide patients and families with a written discharge plan of care in advance of discharge. The plan should reflect collaboration among all disciplines involved in the care of the patient and include information necessary about follow-up services, such as wound care, nutrition, social work, home health nursing, transportation, or any other type of referral. The perioperative nurse also must ensure that documentation is complete regarding any aspects related to the discharge plan of care for which he or she is responsible, including reporting of critical lab values; medical condition and nursing diagnoses; or hand off.

Communication Theories and Techniques, Interviewing Techniques

Effective communication is essential to developing a discharge plan of care among members of the health care team and between the team and patient/family. The perioperative nurse must listen actively and without bias to information the patient and family is providing in order to assess needs completely, relying on interviewing techniques that are appropriate for the situation. If communication barriers exist, those must be addressed first, such as the need for a language interpreter or equipment for patients who are hard of hearing or deaf. If other barriers exist, such as fatigue, depression, cultural issues, or distractions, these must be accounted for as the plan is developed. Communication among caregivers also is important, and the perioperative nurse must be committed to obtaining and sharing information, being an advocate for the patient/family, and involving other disciplines to create the most effective discharge plan of care possible.

Quality Improvement Principles

Quality improvement principles are described well elsewhere in this study guide. Some key points to consider when evaluating the quality of discharge planning are:

- how well are identified outcomes achieved;
- how well is the plan of care communicated between disciplines;
- how thoroughly is the discharge plan documented;
- do patients and families express satisfaction with the discharge planning process; and
- how unexpected outcomes are addressed, and is there a mechanism for those outcomes to be incorporated into future discharge planning.

The focus of quality improvement may vary depending on the facility's strategic plan and goals, but it must include various aspects related to the discharge planning process.

Responsibilities Regarding Impaired and/or Disruptive Behavior (e.g., patient/family, multidisciplinary health care team members)

The problem of impaired practitioners and their disruptive behavior is discussed in depth elsewhere in this text, and the general considerations apply here as well. For the purposes of discharge planning, impaired or disruptive behavior on the part of the patient or family can have a major effect on the plan of care. Impaired or disruptive behaviors appear in many nursing diagnoses that may apply to the patient undergoing an operative or invasive procedure, including impaired adjustment, anxiety, death anxiety, disturbed body image, impaired verbal communication, dysfunctional family processes, alcoholism, ineffective health maintenance, and a host of other problem diagnoses. Regardless of the problem(s) identified, they must be incorporated into the plan of care, with specific accommodations made to address or compensate for them. For example, the patient or family who are overwhelmed by anxiety will need assistance in managing it before specific components of the discharge plan of care can be understood. As a patient advocate, the perioperative nurse can assess information about impairments and disruptive behavior patterns and incorporate it into an appropriate discharge plan.

Summary

The purpose of discharge planning is to assist the patient and family in moving along the continuum of care toward the ultimate goal of achieving an optimal level of function. Effective discharge planning for the patient undergoing an operative or invasive procedure is an evolving process, starting when the patient agrees to undergo the procedure and ending when recovery is complete. The perioperative nurse contributes to the discharge plan of care by identifying appropriate desired outcomes related to the patient and the procedure. The nurse must collaborate with other members of the health care team to help the patient and family achieve those outcomes as fully as possible. Appropriate and effective discharge planning contributes meaningfully to the health status of the patient and family, and is a clear responsibility of every perioperative nurse.

Case Studies/Discussion Points

In each case study that follows, effective discharge planning must account for the following points:

1. When should discharge planning begin?
2. What goals should be addressed in the discharge plan of care, and how can they be approached in a multidisciplinary manner?
3. What things may affect the postoperative course and discharge, such as the procedure, the patient's health status, and lifestyle considerations?
4. How can the patient/family participate in the rehabilitation process most effectively?
5. What are the specific educational needs associated with the clinical scenario?

Case Study 1

PZ, a 55-year-old woman, is scheduled to undergo repair of a torn left rotator cuff as an ambulatory procedure. She is the sole caretaker for her frail, elderly mother who lives with her, and she states that it is important to both of them that her mother remain at home.

PZ injured her shoulder assisting her mother with routine activities of daily living (ADL) and delayed seeing a surgeon because of her caretaker responsibilities. As a consequence, she is quite uncomfortable and rates the level of her pain as an 8 on a scale of 0 to 10. She is looking forward to having the repair done so she can regain lost function and reduce or eliminate her shoulder pain, but she worries about how her recovery will affect her ability to care for her mother.

PZ is five feet tall and weighs 165 pounds. She smokes one pack of cigarettes per day and was diagnosed a year ago with obstructive sleep apnea (OSA). PZ reports that she has difficulty wearing the continuous positive airway pressure (CPAP) mask that she was given when her OSA was diagnosed. She also has elevated blood pressure, but is managed on medication. She reports that she can become sleepy during the day and often must take naps.

Discussion Points for Case Study 1

1. When should discharge planning begin?

   Discharge planning should begin for PZ in the surgeon's office when she agrees to have her rotator cuff repaired. Her OSA diagnosis is significant because it may affect her ability to have the procedure done on an ambulatory basis. As OSA is diagnosed more frequently and its potential implications are understood more clearly, these patients often must be monitored in the hospital overnight to prevent poor outcomes. The surgeon's office staff may need to work with PZ's insurer to obtain precertification for admission to avoid possible cancellation of her procedure.

   Regardless of her OSA diagnosis, PZ's discharge planning should begin in the surgeon's office so she can be educated about all phases of her perioperative care.

2. What goals should be addressed in the discharge plan of care, and how can they be approached in a multidisciplinary manner?

   PZ's main goals for discharge planning would include pain management and optimal recovery from the procedure as well as ensuring that her mother's care is addressed. She must understand normal responses to a rotator cuff repair and anything that might specifically affect her own recovery. PZ is overweight, and nutritional counseling could be beneficial, although the perioperative nurse could choose to collaborate with other caregivers to ensure this becomes part of the overall discharge plan of care rather than addressing it in the immediate perioperative period. PZ also must understand basic principles of her medication management so that her pain can be controlled as effectively as possible and she takes any other medications correctly, especially her antihypertensives throughout the perioperative period. Lastly, PZ must participate fully in the rehabilitation process to ensure that the operative procedure yields the most benefits possible. These goals must be addressed by a variety of caregivers, including physicians, nutritionists, social workers, and nurses.

3. What factors may affect the postoperative course and discharge, such as the procedure, the patient's health status, and lifestyle considerations?

   PZ's diagnosis of OSA may affect whether she is admitted for an overnight stay after the operative procedure. She also has other health concerns such as hypertension and excess weight, which increase her risk for cardiac disease along with the OSA. Clearly, her mother's dependence on PZ affects her lifestyle and must be addressed so that she can be away from home for the procedure and also so that she can recover and regain shoulder function. The procedure will affect PZ's ability to care for herself as well as her mother; therefore, a plan of care to address these needs must be developed. If PZ's OSA is not effectively treated by the CPAP mask she has, an effective discharge plan must address that as well so she can improve her overall state of health.

4. How can the patient/family participate in the rehabilitation process most effectively?

   PZ must be an active participant in her own rehabilitation, so it is important to include her in setting realistic goals. She will gain the most benefit from the rotator cuff repair if her mother's needs for care are addressed in a way that supports healing. This may mean that the discharge plan includes home care for the mother or a short-term admission to an extended care facility so that PZ can focus on her own recovery needs. The nurse may explore this with the patient at any point during the perioperative phase and then involve other disciplines as appropriate to meet this need.

5. What are the specific educational needs associated with the clinical scenario?

   The educational needs associated with PZ's situation are primarily focused on pain management, wound healing, and regaining of function. PZ needs to understand what to expect in terms of normal pain levels after rotator cuff repair, how to use medications most effectively, nonpharmacologic approaches to managing pain, and realistic expectations for long-term pain control in light of the repair performed on her shoulder. She also needs to understand the basic principles of wound healing so she can support the healing process and minimize her risk of developing a postoperative infection. Part of the wound healing process for PZ will be regaining function in her shoulder, so she must clearly understand any prescribed postoperative exercises and the need for physical therapy after the procedure.

Case Study 2

RM is a 55-year-old man who is scheduled to have an Achilles tendon repair and metaphalangeal fusion to be performed on his left foot after experiencing increasing pain over the past two years. RM lives at home with his wife of 30 years and has two adult children who live in the vicinity and are actively involved in the family. He is in good health except for a cardiac history positive for myocardial infarction (MI) at ages 50 and 52, after which an internal cardioverter defibrillator (ICD) was implanted. RM has had no MIs since the implant and describes himself as being generally in good health. His wife expresses some concern over the possible effect surgery and anesthesia will have on his heart, but acknowledges that his foot pain needs to be surgically addressed so he can gain relief. RM will be admitted to the hospital overnight after the procedure.

Discussion Points for Case Study 2

1. When should discharge planning begin?

   Discharge planning should begin in the surgeon's office when RM decides to proceed with the operative procedure. It is important to gather information about his ICD implant and share that with all caregivers who will be involved in his care so that appropriate arrangements can be made. These arrangements may include having a health care industry representative or someone from the electrophysiology department present at the time of the surgery to manage the device, and sufficient lead time must be allowed for this to take place. There also may be a need to have RM admitted to a monitored bed postoperatively to ensure that the ICD is working properly afterward.

2. What goals should be addressed in the discharge plan of care, and how can they be approached in a multidisciplinary manner?

   RM's goals for discharge planning must address his mobility needs, pain management, wound management, and cardiac status. It is important for him to understand how his mobility will be affected and what can be done to compensate for alterations to his mobility. He also needs to be educated about the pain that is associated with this type of procedure and some effective ways to manage it. As with any invasive procedure, good wound care is important and will greatly affect how RM heals from his procedure. The nurse can play a central role in identifying components of the discharge plan to address all of these issues.

   Also, because of RM's cardiac history and ICD, the discharge plan of care must address potential cardiac issues, including any postoperative follow-up care. Concerns that RM's wife has expressed about how the anesthetic and surgery may affect his heart must be answered directly and completely. The perioperative nurse may collaborate with the anesthesia care provider and surgeon, and also may involve staff from the electrophysiology department and/or the health care industry representative.

3. What factors may affect the postoperative course and discharge, such as the procedure, the patient's health status, and lifestyle considerations?

   RM has a good support system with his wife and adult children living nearby, which have a positive effect on his discharge planning and recovery. His lifestyle doesn't present any problems for the discharge plan to address, as his health status is otherwise good; his cardiac history and ICD, however, are key considerations. RM and his wife must receive the usual procedure-related education to promote recovery and optimal surgical outcomes.

4. How can the patient/family participate in the rehabilitation process most effectively?

   RM and his wife can participate in this process most effectively by involving themselves as much as possible throughout the perioperative phase. They should be receptive to information being presented by all their care givers, including physicians, nurses, physical therapists and others, and they must ask for clarification about any information that is not clear to them. They can prioritize RM's healing by making any necessary accommodations to their home before the procedure or his return home. They can involve their children as an extended support system. They need to understand all they can about pain and medication management and also obtain information about wound care. They also must involve RM's cardiac care provider(s) in advance of the procedure and become knowledgeable about the implications surgery and anesthesia may have on his health status. If they have any preferences about how to participate in the rehabilitation process and their choices can be respected, the perioperative nurse should allow this to occur or communicate it to other members of the health care team.

5. What are the specific educational needs associated with the clinical scenario?

   The specific educational needs for RM are much the same as they would be for many other patients undergoing this procedure, but the perioperative nurse must individualize how the needs are met. RM and his wife must learn about pain management techniques that include both medication and non-pharmacologic therapies. They also must be educated about normal responses to the surgical procedure, as well as unexpected outcomes and what to do should they occur. RM and his wife must learn about limitations to his mobility during the recovery phase and what they can do to safely maintain his ability to perform activities of daily living. They also must be educated about any postoperative follow-up care from a cardiac standpoint. RM and his wife may express preferences as to how they are taught and this should be respected whenever possible.

Suggested Learning Activities

The following learning activities may be helpful in validating your own level of competency in discharge planning and in providing materials to improve your knowledge and skills.

- Review the current AORN Competency Statements in Perioperative Nursing, AORN Standards of Perioperative Clinical Practice, and AORN Outcome Standards for Perioperative Patient Outcomes.

- Review age-specific and transculturally sensitive patient education literature.

- Become aware of pertinent state (e.g., department of public health), national (e.g., JCAHO), and federal (e.g., Centers for Medicare and Medicaid Services) regulatory requirements related to discharge planning.

- Review facility-specific standards of care and programs related to discharge planning.

- Develop awareness of the roles of other members of the multidisciplinary health care team and of community resources.

- Conduct a self-assessment of one's own strengths and opportunities for growth in regard to discharge planning, and then validate this assessment with respected peers.

Chapter 6

Cleaning, Disinfecting, Packaging, and Sterilizing

Darin M. Prescott, RN-BC, BSN, CNOR, CASC

The role of the registered nurse in providing a clean and safe surgical environment has expanded throughout the history of nursing, paralleled with an increased knowledge base, as well as advancements in technology. Today, the perioperative registered nurse is faced with an increased challenge to maintain a clean environment and sterile field for the surgical patient. Regulatory agencies and accrediting bodies continue to focus efforts on reducing surgical infections, thereby promoting positive patient outcomes. The cleaning, disinfecting, packaging, and sterilization of surgical instrumentation and supplies are paramount to infection control and patient safety. The perioperative registered nurse is accountable in these processes that are implemented to prevent infection and provide the safest possible environment for surgical intervention. In addition, the surgical conscience is an integral part of the perioperative registered nurse's role in these processes. This chapter serves as a guideline for content review specific to the role of the perioperative registered nurse in the cleaning, disinfecting, packaging, and sterilizing of surgical instruments and equipment.

Learning Objectives

Individuals preparing for the CNOR exam should direct their study activities toward obtaining the knowledge and skills required to appropriately clean, disinfect, package, and sterilize surgical instruments and equipment. Upon completion of this chapter, the individual should be able to:

1. Identify appropriate sterilization methods.

2. Describe the role of the perioperative registered nurse in ensuring surgical instrumentation, devices, and supplies are properly disinfected and sterilized.

3. List the perioperative registered nurse's role and responsibility in selecting and using appropriate methods for the cleaning, packaging, sterilization, and disinfection of surgical instrumentation, devices, and supplies.

Regulatory Standards and Voluntary Guidelines

Standards and recommended practices are developed in accordance with government, regulatory agency, and expert organizations. Examples of these organizations include the Association of periOperative Registered Nurses (AORN), Association for the Advancement of Medical Instrumentation (AAMI), Joint Commission on Accreditation of Healthcare Organizations (JCAHO), Occupational Safety and Health Administration (OSHA), and the Environmental Protection Agency (EPA). These organizations provide specific guidelines that are synthesized into recommended practices and guidelines. Their research and evidence-based practices are the foundation for many of our policy and procedures. Their parameters guide the practice of the perioperative registered nurse.

Aseptic Technique

Aseptic technique is a term this is integral to the perioperative environment. Aseptic technique is defined as "practices that restrict microorganisms in the environment and on equipment and supplies and that prevent normal body flora from contamination the surgical wound" (Rothrock, 2003). Aseptic technique, when carried out effectively, will prevent surgical infection and enhance healing and recovery time.

Common organisms that cause infection include:

- *Staphylococci*,
- *Enterococci*,
- *Pseudomonads*,
- *Mycobacterium tuberculosis*, and
- viruses, such as hepatitis B virus (HBV), hepatitis C (HCV), and human immunodeficiency virus (HIV).

In recent years, drug resistant bacteria have evolved into infections such as methicillin-resistant *Staphylococcus aureus* (MRSA) and vancomycin-resistant *enterococci* (VRE). Using standard and transmission-based (enhanced) precautions are paramount when caring for patients. These precautions will protect the patient, caregiver, and surgical team. Standard precautions include:

- hand hygiene/glove use,
- masks/eye protection,
- gowns,

(continued on page 82)

Task/Knowledge/Skill Statements

SELECT CLEANING, PACKAGING, STERILIZING, AND DISINFECTING METHODS

- Aseptic technique
- Instruments, supplies, and equipment relating to surgical procedure
- Environmental factors (e.g., temperature; humidity; air exchange; noise)
- Principles of sterilization and disinfection
- Microbiology and infection control
- Standard and transmission-based precautions
- Professional and regulatory standards (e.g., AORN *Standards, Recommended Practices, and Guidelines;* Association for the Advancement of Medical Instrumentation [AAMI])
- Cleaning, packaging, sterilizing and disinfecting methods
- Disinfection procedures for equipment and instruments
- Documentation of sterilization, biological and chemical monitoring
- Selecting cleaning, packaging, sterilizing and disinfecting methods
- Performing and documenting disinfection procedures for equipment and instrument
- Monitoring and documenting package integrity (e.g., tissue; skin; bone; temperature)
- Basic management techniques and delegation
- Regulatory standards and voluntary guidelines (e.g., AORN *Standards, Recommended Practices and Guidelines;* OSHA; JCAHO; ANA Code of Ethics for Nurses with Explications for Perioperative Nurses; state Nurse Practice Act)
- Nursing research and evidence-based practice

PERFORM ENVIRONMENTAL CLEANING (E.G., SPILLS; ROOM TURN OVER; TERMINAL CLEANING)

- Surgical procedure
- Aseptic technique
- Principles of sterilization disinfection
- Microbiology and infection control
- Standard and transmission-based precautions
- Professional and regulatory standards (e.g., AORN *Standards, Recommended Practices, and Guidelines;* Association for the Advancement of Medical Instrumentation [AAMI])
- Environmental cleaning (e.g., spills; room turnover; terminal cleaning)
- Disinfection procedures for equipment and instruments
- Handling and disposing of hazardous materials (e.g., chemo drugs; CJD, needles; sharps)
- Performing environmental cleaning (e.g., spills; room turnover; terminal cleaning)
- Environmental hazards, disasters, preparedness, and response (e.g., fire; toxic fumes; natural disasters; terrorism)
- Regulatory standards and voluntary guidelines (e.g., AORN *Standards, Recommended Practices and Guidelines;* OSHA; JCAHO; ANA Code of Ethics for Nurses with Explications for Perioperative Nurses; state Nurse Practice Act)

PERFORM AND DOCUMENT DISINFECTION PROCEDURES FOR EQUIPMENT AND INSTRUMENTS

- Surgical procedure
- Aseptic technique
- Instruments, supplies, and equipment relating to surgical procedure
- Documentation of all nursing interventions
- Standard and transmission-based precautions
- Professional and regulatory standards (e.g., AORN *Standards, Recommended Practices, and Guidelines;* Association for the Advancement of Medical Instrumentation [AAMI])
- Cleaning, packaging, sterilizing and disinfecting methods
- Disinfection procedures for equipment and instruments
- Documentation of sterilization, biological and chemical monitoring
- Selecting cleaning, packaging, sterilizing and disinfecting methods
- Performing and documenting disinfection procedures for equipment and instruments
- Performing and documenting sterilization procedures
- Conducting and documenting biological monitoring
- Conducting and documenting chemical monitoring
- Principles of equipment inspection and maintenance

HANDLE AND DISPOSE OF HAZARDOUS MATERIALS (E.G., CHEMO DRUGS; CJD; NEEDLES; SHARPS)

- Surgical procedure
- Principles of patient safety
- Aseptic technique
- Instruments, supplies, and equipment relating to surgical procedure
- Microbiology and infection control
- Standard and transmission-based precautions
- Professional and regulatory standards (e.g., AORN *Standards, Recommended Practices, and Guidelines,* Association for the Advancement of Medical Instrumentation [AAMI])
- Environmental cleaning (e.g., spills; room turnover; terminal cleaning)
- Handling and disposing of hazardous materials (e.g., chemo drugs; CJD, needles; sharps)
- Performing environmental cleaning (e.g., spills, room turnover; terminal cleaning)

→

Task/Knowledge/Skill Statements

- Handling and disposing of hazardous materials (e.g., chemo drugs; CJD)
- Environmental hazards, disasters, preparedness, and response (e.g., fire; toxic fumes; natural disasters; terrorism)
- Quality improvement principles
- Regulatory standards and voluntary guidelines (e.g., AORN *Standards, Recommended Practices and Guidelines*; OSHA; JCHAO; ANA Code of Ethics for Nurses with Explications for Perioperative Nurses; state Nurse Practice Act)
- Nursing research and evidence-based practice

PERFORM AND DOCUMENT STERILIZATION PROCEDURES

- Surgical procedure
- Aseptic technique
- Instruments, supplies, and equipment relating to surgical procedure
- Implants (e.g., handling; tracking; sterilization)
- Documentation of all nursing interventions
- Principles of sterilization disinfection
- Professional and regulatory standards (e.g., AORN *Standards, Recommended Practices, and Guidelines,* Association for the Advancement of Medical Instrumentation [AAMI])
- Cleaning, packaging, sterilizing and disinfecting methods
- Disinfection procedures for equipment and instruments
- Documentation of sterilization, biological and chemical monitoring
- Selecting cleaning, packaging, sterilizing and disinfecting methods
- Performing and documenting disinfection procedures for equipment and instruments
- Performing and documenting sterilization procedures
- Conducting and documenting biological monitoring
- Conducting and documenting chemical monitoring
- Quality improvement principles
- Monitoring and documenting package integrity (e.g., tissue; skin; bone; temperature)
- Regulatory standards and voluntary guidelines (e.g., AORN *Standards, Recommended Practices and Guidelines*; OSHA; JCHAO; ANA Code of Ethics for Nurses with Explications for Perioperative nurses; state Nurse Practice Act)

CONDUCT AND DOCUMENT BIOLOGICAL MONITORING

- Surgical procedure
- Aseptic technique
- Instruments, supplies, and equipment relating to surgical procedure
- Documentation of all nursing interventions
- Principles of sterilization disinfection
- Professional and regulatory standards (e.g., AORN *Standards, Recommended Practices, and Guidelines,* Association for the Advancement of Medical Instrumentation [AAMI])
- Cleaning, packaging, sterilizing and disinfecting methods
- Disinfection procedures for equipment and instruments
- Documentation of sterilization, biological and chemical monitoring
- Performing and documenting disinfection procedures for equipment and instruments
- Performing and documenting sterilization procedures
- Conducting and documenting biological monitoring
- Quality improvement principles
- Monitoring and documenting package integrity (e.g., tissue; skin; bone; temperature)
- Regulatory standards and voluntary guidelines (e.g., AORN *Standards, Recommended Practices and Guidelines*; OSHA; JCHAO; ANA Code of Ethics for Nurses with Explications for Perioperative Nurses; state Nurse Practice Act)

CONDUCT AND DOCUMENT MONITORING OF CHEMICAL DISINFECTANTS AND/OR STERILANTS

- Surgical procedure
- Aseptic technique
- Instruments, supplies, and equipment relating to surgical procedure
- Documentation of all nursing interventions
- Principles of sterilization disinfection
- Professional and regulatory standards (e.g., AORN *Standards, Recommended Practices, and Guidelines,* Association for the Advancement of Medical Instrumentation [AAMI])
- Cleaning, packaging, sterilizing and disinfecting methods
- Disinfection procedures for equipment and instruments
- Documentation of sterilization, biological and chemical monitoring
- Performing and documenting disinfection procedures for equipment and instruments
- Performing and documenting sterilization procedures
- Conducting and documenting chemical monitoring
- Quality improvement principles
- Monitoring and documenting package integrity (e.g., tissue; skin; bone; temperature)
- Regulatory standards and voluntary guidelines (e.g., AORN *Standards, Recommended Practices and Guidelines*; OSHA; JCHAO; ANA Code of Ethics for Nurses with Explications for Perioperative Nurses; state Nurse Practice Act)

(continued from page 79)

- appropriate sharps handling, and
- environmental procedures including patient care equipment and linen handling, environmental control, and patient placement.

Enhanced precautions are the second tier of precautions that are used for patients with identified or suspected infectious processes with highly transmissible or epidemiologically important pathogens. These precautions include:

- airborne precautions,
- droplet precautions,
- contact precautions, and
- providing a protective environment.

Cleaning, Packaging, Sterilizing, Disinfecting Methods, Creutzfeldt-Jakob Disease (CJD)

The perioperative registered nurse has the accountability for ensuring that interventions maintain the highest standard with regard to the cleaning, packaging, sterilization, and disinfection of surgical instruments, devices, and supplies. As an overseer of the surgical team, the perioperative registered nurse holds accountability with regard to surgical conscience and the maintenance of aseptic technique in the preoperative and intraoperative phases.

Cleaning

Recommended practices exist to provide a general guideline for the care of instrumentation. However, manufacturers' instructions provide specific direction for the care, cleaning, handling, and use of surgical instruments and powered equipment. Decontamination of surgical instrumentation takes place after each patient use or in the event of contamination. It is required before sterilization or high level disinfection. "Decontamination is defined as the process of eliminating many or all pathogenic organisms except bacterial spores from inanimate objects." (Rothrock, 2003).

Cleaning of surgical instruments consists of presoaking or prerinsing to prevent bioburden from drying on instruments or to soften dried on debris. This may be accomplished by soaking in a covered basin with demineralized distilled water and a low-sudsing detergent. Commercial enzymatic spray detergents also are available in liquid or foam consistencies that may be sprayed on instruments without the use of water.

In the decontamination of surgical instrumentation, automated and/or manual cleaning methods are indicated. Automated methods include washer/sterilizers, ultrasonic cleaners, and washer/decontaminators. Manual cleaning may be performed with appropriate use of personal protective equipment (PPE). The following recommended practice points must be considered.

- Powered equipment and any attachments should be decontaminated and disassembled before decontamination.
- Inspection and check for functionality should be completed after decontamination and before storage.
- Instruments should be kept free of gross soil during surgical procedures by wiping with a sponge moistened with sterile water.
- Sterile water should be used in the irrigation of lumened instrumentation. Saline causes deterioration and should not be used for cleaning or irrigation.
- All instruments on the sterile field require decontamination.
- PPE should be worn throughout the intraoperative phase and decontamination process.
- Policies and procedures should be reviewed periodically and made available in the practice setting.

The perioperative registered nurse's responsibilities regarding cleaning of surgical instruments and medical devices ensure that:

- manufacturers' instructions are followed with regard to cleaning, handling, and sterilization;
- instruments are kept free of gross soiling during surgical and invasive procedures;
- decontamination is performed in a manner that minimizes risk to those performing the task;
- automated devices are utilized whenever possible to process instruments and manual cleaning is accomplished using appropriate PPE;
- transportation of soiled instruments takes place in a covered container with water to ease the removal of bioburden; and
- appropriate disinfection solutions are used at the acceptable level according to manufacturers' recommendations.

Packaging

Packaging systems used by the perioperative registered nurse should meet the manufacturers' guidelines and also be compatible with the sterilization method being used. Packaging systems may include woven fabric, non-woven materials, peel pouches (synthetic and paper), and container systems. Packaging systems must maintain the sterility of their contents until the package is opened. They should also allow for aseptic presentation of the contents to the sterile field without contamination. Peel packages should be used according to manufacturers' recommendations. The following recommended practice points should be considered.

- Packaging systems should be evaluated according to

the current AORN Recommended Practices for Selection and Use of Packaging Systems and Product Selection in Perioperative Practice Settings.
- Packaging systems should be compatible with the sterilization process being considered.

The perioperative registered nurse's responsibilities regarding packaging ensure that:

- the system used is appropriate based on item size and type;
- the system has an outside indication that sterilization has occurred as well as an internal indicator;
- no breaks in packaging have occurred (e.g., missing breakaway locks; missing or improperly used filters; holes, tears, or water spots);
- a label identifying the lot control number and identification of the assembler is in place;
- policies and procedures are readily available and followed within the practice setting; and
- the cost analysis is appropriate to the method of packaging.

Sterilizing

Sterilization is defined as "the complete elimination or destruction of all forms of microbial life" (Rothrock, 2003). Sterilization may be accomplished through various methods in the perioperative setting. Sterilizer and instrument manufacturers' instructions for exposure times and temperature settings should be followed to ensure sterilization is achieved. Each sterilizer load must contain a sterilization process monitoring device.

Steam sterilization is by far the oldest, safest, most economic, and well understood method of sterilization for items that can withstand heat and moisture. Steam sterilization may be accomplished with packaged items or flashed items. Three factors are required for steam sterilization: time, temperature, and moisture. The two most common types of sterilizers used in the perioperative setting are gravity displacement and prevacuum. Gravity, as it implies, allows steam to penetrate the chamber based on gravity of the steam from the top downward. Prevacuum draws the steam downward and displaces air much faster than gravity.

The Association for the Advancement of Medical Instrumentation (AAMI) recommends that the temperature settings for loads with porous or nonporous items in the gravity displacement sterilizer be at (AORN, 2006):

- 250° F (121° C) for exposure times of 30 minutes; or
- 270° F (132° C) for exposure times of 15 or 25 minutes; or
- 275° F (135° C) for exposure times of 10 minutes.

For autoclaves with prevacuum capability, temperatures should reach:

- 270° F (132° C) for exposure times of 4 minutes; or
- 275° F (135° C) for exposure times of 3 minutes.

Cooling, drying, and storing are remaining components of steam sterilized items.

Flash sterilization times differ from packaged items. AAMI recommends that temperature settings for both the gravity displacement and prevacuum sterilizers should be 270-272° F. (132-135° C). The minimum exposure time for metal or nonporous items is 3 minutes. If the load consists of metal items with lumens and porous items (e.g., rubber, plastic) to be sterilized together, the exposure time required is 10 minutes in a gravity cycle and 4 minutes in a prevacuum cycle. Flash sterilization should only be considered in clinical situations if the following parameters are met:

- there is not adequate time to package and sterilize the item(s) in a full cycle;
- instruments have been decontaminated, inspected, and disassembled into a mesh bottom tray;
- sterilizer function has been tested daily with a biological indicator;
- sterilizer function is monitored with each load;
- the sterilizer is located in a proximity that allows for aseptic delivery of the sterilized instruments to the sterile field;
- safety devices are available to transfer hot and heavy trays to the sterile field; and
- aseptic technique is maintained during transfer of the item(s) from the autoclave to the sterile field.

Implants

Sterilization of implants is a priority of the perioperative registered nurse caring for patients who will have these devices implanted. Implantable devices, which are frequently processed outside of the manufacturer, may include items such as plates, screws, femoral rods, and wire. Manufacturers' written instructions are to be followed with all decontamination, packaging, and sterilization processes. A biological indicator should be included in each load that contains implantable devices. AAMI recommends that these items be quarantined until the outcome of the biological indicator has proven that the sterilization cycle was effective. By monitoring the parameters of time, temperature, and pressure, risk of sterilization failure can be diminished.

Flash sterilization is not indicated for implantable items. Adequate planning should provide for an adequate supply of properly sterilized implantable items. The AORN

Recommended Practices for Sterilization in the Perioperative Practice Setting state that flash sterilization should not be used for implantable devices (AORN, 2006). However, if an implant must be flashed in an emergency situation, a rapid-action biological monitoring device should be used, along with a class V chemical integrator. The implant should not be released for use until a negative result from the rapid-action biological indicator is obtained. After the negative result is obtained, the implant may be released for immediate use. If the implant is not used, it cannot be resterilized for future use.

Alternative Sterilization Methods

There are alternative sterilization methods for heat- and moisture-sensitive surgical instruments and equipment. Ethylene oxide (EO) is a one sterilization method used for these types of sensitive surgical items. Key considerations with regard to EO sterilizer use include following the manufacturers' recommendations for mechanical aeration to remove the EO from the items sterilized and monitoring for occupational exposure of employees.

Low-temperature gas plasma sterilization also may be used for moisture-stable, moisture-sensitive, and heat-sensitive items. Plasma sterilization may replace EO sterilization in many areas. It allows for a significantly less turnaround time and does not require aeration. Non-woven and polypropylene wraps and pouches must be used in gas plasma sterilization, due to vapor absorption of hydrogen peroxide activation.

Peracetic acid is a low temperature sterilization process used for immersible surgical instrument and/or equipment for just-in-time use. Items sterilized in an automated system using peracetic acid should be used immediately, as items immersed cannot be packaged. Therefore, careful attention must be paid to indicators and continuity of the item(s) once the sterilization process is completed until the time of use. Manufacturers' recommendations must be followed with regard to the device used to sterilize with peracetic acid and the items being sterilized. In addition, quality controls must be established and include:

- sterilizer maintenance history;
- sterilization process monitoring by biological, chemical, or mechanical devices;
- air removal testing (e.g., Bowie-Dick test) for prevacuum sterilizers;
- lot control and traceability of load contents;
- orientation, continuing education, and trending records; and
- sterilization cycle information including control number, contents, exposure times, temperatures, operator name, and results.

Disinfecting Methods

Disinfection is defined as "the process of eliminating many or all pathogenic organisms except bacterial spores from inanimate objects" (Rothrock, 2003). Disinfectants are classified as high-, intermediate-, or low-level. Items to be disinfected should be categorized as critical, semicritical, and noncritical. The Spaulding classification system is used by practitioners to determine the correct processing methods for preparing instruments and other items for patient use. Critical items are those that enter sterile tissue or the vascular system and should be sterile when used (e.g., surgical instruments, implants, needles). Semicritical items are those that come in contact with nonintact skin or mucous membranes (e.g., bronchoscopes, gastrointestinal scopes, anesthesia equipment). High-level disinfection may be appropriate for these items. Noncritical items that come in contact with intact skin only (e.g., blood pressure cuffs, OR furnishings) are disinfected with an intermediate- or low-level disinfectant.

High-level disinfection products are available in a liquid form to immerse items for semicritical use. Manufacturers' recommendations must be followed for the use and handling of these products. Testing methods must be used to ensure the liquid is at a level to achieve high level disinfection with a test determined by the manufacturer. All lumens must be irrigated with the high-level disinfection solution and rinsed with sterile water upon completion of the manufacturers' recommended exposure time.

Chemical disinfectant vapors may present environmental challenges. The OSHA guidelines for exposure, as well as for discarding expired solution, must be followed. In recent years, a number of products that do not require ventilation have become available. Because this is a liquid product, PPE, including eye protection, is necessary for safe handling. Written policies should be developed regarding the transportation of high-level disinfected items from the disinfection area to the place of use. Quality control programs must also be in place to address:

- documentation of date, time, type of disinfectant, test results prior to use, temperature of the disinfectant, load contents, submersion time, and patient identifier;
- orientation and continued competency; and
- quality control checks and monitoring of solution replacement intervals.

Creutzfeldt-Jakob Disease

Creutzfeldt-Jakob disease (CJD) is a rare and fatal disease of the nervous system. The prion that causes CJD is an isoform of normal protein concentrated in brain tissue. Prions are generally resistant to standard sterilization procedures including steam, EO, and high-level disinfection. Tissues vary with regard to their infectivity depending on prion content. High-infectivity tissue includes central nervous system tissue, brain dura mater, spinal cord, and corneal tissue. Medium-infectivity includes body fluid and tissue such as cerebrospinal fluid, lymph nodes, spleen, and pituitary gland. Low-infectivity includes body fluid and tissue such as blood, bone marrow, heart, lung, liver, kidney, thyroid, skin, prostate, semen, placenta, vaginal secretions, breast milk, tears, and mucous.

Surgical instruments require special consideration when making decisions during the decontamination phase.

- Disposable items should be used as much as possible, including instrumentation and supplies.
- Low-infectivity items should be kept separate and moist between the time of exposure and subsequent decontamination and cleaning.
- After thorough cleaning, if the item is heat tolerant, steam autoclave at 272° F (134° C) for 18 minutes in a prevacuum sterilizer or 250° F (121° C) for 60 minutes in a gravity sterilizer.
- Items may be soaked for 60 minutes in a 1 Normal sodium hydroxide solution. After one hour, rinse, clean, and sterilize as above.
- Items that are impossible to be cleaned should be discarded.
- Use of power saws and drills should be avoided as their design is difficult to clean and too expensive to discard.

Perform Environmental Cleaning

The perioperative registered nurse is accountable for environmental cleaning as part of maintaining a safe, clean environment. Although this function often is delegated to unlicensed assistive personnel, the nurse is accountable for ensuring that the facility policies and procedures for environmental cleaning are executed. Cleaning should be performed on a regular basis to reduce the amount of dust, organic debris, and microbial load in surgical environments. Operating rooms should be cleaned before and after each surgical procedure and terminally cleaned at the end of the day.

Spills

Spills outside of the surgical field should be cleaned up as soon as possible. When cleaning spills of blood or other potentially infections material, use appropriate PPE. Small spills are defined as less than 10 mL and should be cleaned using a soft, absorbent, low-linting cloth and either an intermediate level germicide (i.e., an EPA-registered germicide that possesses a tuberculocidal claim or having a label claim for HIV and/or HBV). Sodium hypochlorite (i.e., chlorine bleach) in a 1:100 dilution may be used for small spills on nonporous surfaces. For large spills, those more than 10 mL, blood and other potentially infections material should be cleaned first using a disposable absorbent material, followed by application of the selected germicidal product. Materials used for cleaning should be discarded in biohazard containers. For large spills, a 1:10 dilution of sodium hypochlorite may be added to the spill before cleanup.

It is recommended that a fresh solution of sodium hypochlorite for cleaning and disinfection be prepared daily for maximum effectiveness. Because this solution may cause pitting of surgical instruments and metal surfaces, it is preferable to have an EPA-registered, hospital-grade tuberculocidal product available. Inanimate porous objects that become contaminated should be discarded and replaced or handled accordingly.

Discarding Sharps and Infectious Materials

Sharps include disposable needles, scalpels, staplers, and electrosurgical tips. All sharps should be discarded in appropriate puncture-resistant containers that are labeled or tagged for easy identification as biohazardous waste. Contaminated items are placed in leak-proof containers or color-coded bags to prevent exposing personnel to blood, tissue, and/or body fluids, as well as to prevent contamination of the surgical environment. Containers should be changed as directed by facility policy.

Room Turn Over

Reusable items (i.e., instruments and supplies) should be transported out of the OR for decontamination and reprocessing using covered washable carts. Patient transport vehicles, OR equipment, and furniture that are visibly soiled should be cleaned with a hospital-grade germicidal agent at the end of each surgical procedure. Walls, doors, surgical lights, and ceilings should be spot cleaned as needed. Floors should be cleaned if visibly soiled using a freshly laundered or new mop head with hospital-grade germicidal agent in a 3- to 4-foot perimeter around the OR bed. The mop head should be dipped only once into the solution and not redipped into the same solution. If the used mop head is redipped into the same solution, the solution must be discarded and replaced. The OR bed should be moved to check for contamination and debris during room turn over.

Terminal Cleaning

Operating rooms, regardless of use, should be terminally cleaned during each 24-hour period during the regular work week. Mechanical friction and use of an EPA-registered agent are used to clean equipment and areas including, but not limited to:

- surgical lights and fixed and ceiling mounted equipment;
- furniture and equipment, including wheels, casters, step stools, foot pedals, telephones, and light switches;
- hallways and floors;
- handles of cabinets and push plates;
- ventilation face plates;
- horizontal surfaces;
- sub-sterile areas; and
- scrub/utility areas and scrub sinks.

The OR floor should be wet vacuumed with an EPA-registered hospital-grade disinfectant after the last scheduled procedure of the day or at least once in 24 hours. Cleaning equipment should be disassembled, cleaned with a facility approved agent, dried, and stored to prevent microbial growth. In addition, all areas of equipment in the surgical practice area should be cleaned according to an established schedule including, but not limited to:

- ducts and filters;
- air-conditioning equipment;
- return ventilation and heating grills;
- recessed ceiling tracks;
- closets, cabinets, and shelves;
- storerooms;
- sterilizers, warming cabinets, refrigerators, ice machines, freezers;
- walls and ceilings; and
- offices, lounges, lavatories, and locker rooms.

Perform and Document Disinfection Procedure for Equipment and Instruments

Documentation of disinfection for equipment and instrumentation is a responsibility of the perioperative registered nurse. The commercial disinfectant used should be registered with the EPA. Label information on the commercial product should include warnings, instructions for use, intended action, and aftercare instructions. Disinfection should take place immediately before use or immediately after contamination. Appropriate PPE, including eye protection, is required when using high-level disinfectants based on the manufacturers' recommendations. Effective cleaning to remove any bioburden is crucial to optimizing the effectiveness of a disinfectant. "A record of the agent and time of exposure should be maintained by the facility as a method to track semi critical items that have undergone high-level disinfection" (Berry & Kohn, 2005). This record should include the following information:

- date;
- solution used and type of agent;
- strength;
- activation date;
- expiration date;
- temperature;
- immersion time in and out; and
- load control number, location, and contents.

Handle and Dispose of Hazardous Materials

Biohazardous waste should be placed in a specifically labeled biohazard leak-proof bag. The bag should then be placed in hard-sided transportation containers that can be cleaned between uses. Prevention of exposure and puncture injuries is a responsibility of the entire surgical team. This prevents a specific risk to the users as well as handlers. Sharps should not be manipulated by hand. Instruments such as heavy hemostats should be used when manipulating scalpel blades and syringe needles. Needle holders should be used to attach a suture needle directly from the packet when possible. Using a neutral zone to transfer sharps on the field alleviates hand-to-hand passing and risk of puncture injury. Syringe needles should never be recapped without the use of a recapping safety device. In the event of a puncture injury:

- remove the puncturing sharp or instrument from the sterile field;
- remove both gloves using the open glove technique;
- squeeze the skin to release the blood;
- wash hands with antiseptic under running water;
- irrigate the wound with a virucidal agent such as iodine, bleach, or peroxide; and
- report the incident per facility policy and complete necessary testing.

Drug disposal at the end of a case should be completed as directed by the policy of the facility including specific local, state, and federal regulations. Specific disposal regimens for drugs such as narcotics or chemo-therapeutic agents must be followed.

Perform and Document Sterilization Procedures

Documentation of sterilization is required of items whether sterilized within the facility or at an outside location. Load control numbers are required and should be imprinted on the package of each sterile item. Various labeling systems exist, such as writing on the package before sterilization, machine-labeling systems, and peel-off bar codes. This method of tracking is used in case recall of the sterilized item is required. Sterility is event-related, unless it contains specific unstable items such as medications or chemicals. Items are considered sterile based on the assumption that handling and storage are within appropriate facility parameters. Rotation of supplies should occur with the newest supplies being rotated with the oldest. Flash sterilization documentation should include the item(s) flash sterilized and that sterilization parameters were met per facility policy.

Conduct and Document Biological Monitoring

As noted, steam sterilization is the most common form of sterilization. Biological monitoring is performed to ensure effectiveness of the sterilizer. For flash sterilizers, a biological indicator is used in the bottom of a tray of instruments and is placed in the lower front of the autoclave. For gravity displacement sterilizers, a test pack with a chemical indicator inside is placed in the lower front of the autoclave. Test packs may be made with linen and supplies within the facility or commercially obtained based on manufacturer recommendations. The significance of the lower front of the autoclave is that this is the coldest point in the autoclave and presents the greatest challenge for steam penetration. The prevacuum sterilizer has the same requirement of a test pack as the gravity displacement sterilizer. In addition, a Bowie-Dick test is run to determine that air is removed from the sterilizer. This test pack is placed on the lower shelf, horizontally over the drain of an empty prevacuum chamber.

Summary

Cleaning, disinfecting, packaging, and sterilizing are significant interventions in the surgical environment. The perioperative registered nurse is accountable for making sure that optimal efforts are made to ensure that these processes are implemented effectively for each and every patient. The perioperative registered nurse serves as a resource for all personnel within the surgical services area. Following manufacturers' recommendations, facility policies and procedures, in conjunction with current standards, recommended practices, and guidelines will enhance patient care and promote positive patient outcomes.

Case Studies/Discussion Points

Case Study 1

You are the circulator, opening a set of instruments for an open reduction and internal fixation of a left ankle. There are three trays of specialty instrumentation including implantable plates and screws for this procedure. All trays are labeled and identified with the same load number. All tape outside of the wrapped trays is turned black, indicating steam exposure. One of the trays does not have a chemical indicator inside of the tray. The other two have chemical indicators present that have turned color, indicating effective steam penetration. The case is scheduled to begin in approximately 30 minutes.

Discussion Points for Case Study 1

- Is there a sterile replacement tray available?
- Can the case be delayed to accommodate the necessary time to reprocess it?
- Can the tray be flash sterilized?
- Is there a risk to the patient if flash sterilization is chosen?
- Can you assume that the instrumentation is sterile based on the other trays having positive indicators and being from the same cycle of the sterilizer?

Responses to consider:

- Planning and coordination will alleviate the need for flash sterilization. This includes scheduling cases appropriately (e.g., not scheduling back-to-back cases requiring the same instrumentation) and ensuring adequate numbers of instruments are available to perform multiple cases without flash sterilizing instruments.

- Delaying the case may present an inconvenience to the patient and surgical team. However, appropriately processing the instrumentation will provide optimal care to the patient. The patient's physical condition will also need to be assessed as to whether waiting is appropriate.

- Flash sterilization is not recommended for implantable devices (e.g., plates and screws).

- There is an increased risk of contamination if flash sterilization is chosen, as there is additional handling to transport the tray from sterilizer to the field.

- You cannot assume that the instrumentation is sterile based on the other trays being from the same cycle of the sterilizer having positive indicators. There is no definitive way to determine that steam reached the inner contents of the tray without an indicator.

Case Study 2

You are the scrub person during a small bowel resection. An additional pan of retractors has been requested. The circulator brings in the wrapped pan of instruments and opens it appropriately on a small table. As you approach the pan, you notice beads of water on the inside of the tray. The chemical indicator is present and color change indicates effective steam penetration. The tray was located on the shelf in its customary location. What are your next actions?

Discussion Points for Case Study 2

- Are the instruments sterile to use?
- What are the ramifications of this load being wet?
- What is the significance of the load cycle lot number in this instance?

Responses to consider:

- Wrapped instruments that are opened and found wet are not considered to be sterile.

- The instruments should be replaced with new instrumentation. If flash sterilization is necessary, the instruments should be decontaminated appropriately first.

- The load cycle lot number will need to be tracked to recall all other wrapped items for possible wetness.

Suggested Learning Activities

- Maintain current knowledge on new methods of cleaning, disinfecting, packaging, and sterilizing surgical instruments, equipment, and supplies.

- Research the literature for related articles.

- Review facility policies and procedures for cleaning, disinfecting, packaging, and sterilizing surgical instruments, equipment, and supplies—recommend updates as needed based on current literature findings.

Chapter 7

Emergency Situations

Rose Moss, RN, MN, CNOR
Charles J. Moss, III, CRNA, MS

The actions of the perioperative nurse in emergency situations, regardless of the nature of the situation, are comparable to his or her responses during all patient care activities, with the exception of time. The Association of periOperative Registered Nurses' (AORN) philosophy statement affirms that nurses must be ethical, responsible, and accountable for quality patient care. Patient undergoing surgery or other invasive procedures have diminished self-care abilities and protective reflexes; therefore, they are vulnerable and require a higher level of nursing care (Simunek, 1996). Because of these inherent characteristics, the perioperative nurse, as the patient's advocate in an emergency situation in the surgical environment, should focus on two primary patient outcomes—keeping the patient free from injury and keeping the patient free from infection.

This chapter provides a review of the perioperative nurse's role in emergency situations, based on the identified task statements and requisite knowledge and skills to perform those tasks. The content of this chapter focuses on the following areas:

- overview of nursing practice issues;
- performing nursing interventions, specifically surgical nursing interventions, cardiopulmonary resuscitation (CPR), and management of a malignant hyperthermia (MH) crisis;
- directing multidisciplinary health care team members; and
- safeguarding patients and members of the health care team from environmental hazards and disasters, such as fire, toxic fumes, natural disasters, and terrorism.

Learning Objectives

Individuals preparing for the CNOR exam will direct their study activities toward obtaining the knowledge and skills required to respond appropriately in emergency situations. Upon completion of this chapter, the individual should be able to:

1. Describe the role of the perioperative nurse during any type of perioperative emergency situation.
2. Outline current legal responsibilities, regulatory standards, and voluntary guidelines related to perioperative nursing actions during emergency situations.
3. Discuss the knowledge and skills required for a perioperative nurse to perform effectively in an emergency situation.
4. Identify appropriate nursing interventions during various patient emergencies.
5. Explain the role of the perioperative nurse as a member of a multidisciplinary team in emergency situations.

Overview of Nursing Practice Issues

Legal Responsibilities and Implications for Patient Care

The practice of professional nursing is a theory-based, goal-directed activity to assist clients in meeting their basic human needs. Assessment, communication, interpersonal relationships, and the nursing process as a clinical decision-making strategy are integral components of the professional nurse's role. Nursing also is influenced by scientific and technological advancements, as well as economic, political, and social forces.

One of the dominant social forces affecting nursing today is the legal climate. The perioperative nurse is in a position of trust and confidence to the surgical patient and therefore has a fiduciary relationship with him or her (Simunek, 1996). The 2006 AORN Competency Statements in Perioperative Nursing state that perioperative nursing care must be delivered within the legal standards of practice. This is especially true in emergency situations that occur during surgery or other invasive procedures. The nurse practice act in each state provides the legal definition of nursing, and the law protects the safety and health of the public by establishing the legal qualifications for who can practice nursing in that state. It is important for every perioperative nurse to know the legal definition of nursing practice as outlined in the state's nurse practice act and to practice within that scope.

Task/Knowledge/Skill Statements

Performing nursing interventions (e.g., surgical; CPR; MH)

- Anatomy and physiology
- Legal responsibilities and implications for patient care
- Surgical procedure
- Pharmacology and anesthetic agents
- Anesthetic interventions (e.g., assist as needed)
- Principles of patient safety
- Physiologic responses to the surgical experience including potential complication
- Principles of positioning
- Documentation of all nursing interventions
- Environmental factors (e.g., temperature; humidity; air exchange; noise)
- Emergency procedures (e.g., surgical; CPR; MH)
- Environmental hazards, disasters, preparedness, and response (e.g., fire; toxic fumes; natural disasters; terrorism)
- Quality improvement principles
- Basic management techniques and delegation
- Nursing research and evidence-based practice

Direct multidisciplinary health care team members

- Legal responsibilities and implications for patient care
- Documentation of all nursing interventions
- Reporting techniques to multidisciplinary health care providers (e.g., critical lab values; medical condition; medications; allergies; implants/implantable devices; hand off; read back verbal orders; communication barriers)
- Postoperative complications
- Emergency procedures (e.g., surgical; CPR; MH)
- Environmental hazards, disasters, preparedness, and response (e.g., fire, toxic fumes; natural disasters; terrorism)
- Basic management techniques and delegation
- Regulatory standards and voluntary guidelines (e.g., AORN *Standards, Recommended Practices, and Guidelines;* OSHA; JCHAO; ANA Code of Ethics for Nurses with Explications for Perioperative Nurses; state Nurse Practice Act)
- Clinical privileges

Safeguard patients and members of the health care team from environmental hazards and disasters (e.g., fire; toxic fumes; natural disasters; terrorism)

- Patient rights and responsibilities
- Legal responsibilities and implications for patient care
- Principles of patient safety
- Ergonomics and body mechanics (e.g., patient/equipment)
- Emergency procedures (e.g., surgical; CPR; MH)
- Environmental hazards, disasters, preparedness, and response (e.g., fire; toxic fumes; natural disasters; terrorism)
- Regulatory standards and voluntary guidelines (e.g., AORN *Standards, Recommended Practices, and Guidelines;* OSHA; JCHAO; ANA Code of Ethics for Nurses with Explications for Perioperative Nurses; state Nurse Practice Act)
- Responsibilities regarding impaired and/or disruptive behavior (e.g., patient/family; multidisciplinary health care team members)
- Nursing research and evidence-based practice

Regulatory Standards and Voluntary Guidelines

There are regulatory standards and voluntary guidelines promulgated by various professional associations, federal agencies, and other organizations that impact the practice of nursing. AORN publishes and its updated *Standards, Recommended Practices, and Guidelines* annually. The purpose of these documents is to provide direction to perioperative nursing practice and a comprehensive approach to meeting surgical patients' health needs.

The Occupational Safety and Health Administration's (OSHA) mission is to ensure the safety and health of America's workers by developing and enforcing standards; providing training, outreach, and education; establishing partnerships; and promoting continual improvement in workplace safety and health. OSHA standards include those related to occupational exposure to bloodborne pathogens and tuberculosis protection. It also provides advisory guidelines for preventing workplace violence for health care and social service workers.

The Joint Commission on Accreditation of Healthcare Organizations (JCAHO) is a regulating body that focuses on patient safety. The Joint Commission addresses standards of care and performance in specific areas. These standards ensure that patients receive care that is provided in a safe manner and in a secure environment.

A panel of patient safety experts oversees the development and annual updating of the JCAHO National Patient Safety Goals (NPSGs). The purpose of the NPSGs is to promote precise improvements in patient safety. The goals highlight problem areas in health care and explain evidence-based and expert-based solutions to these problems. In addition, the goals focus on system-wide solutions where possible, through the recognition that sound system design is intrinsic to the delivery of safe, high quality health care. Briefly, the 2007 Hospital/Critical Access Hospital NPSGs are (JCAHO, 2006):

- Goal 1: Improve the accuracy of patient identification.
- Goal 2: Improve the effectiveness of communication among caregivers.
- Goal 3: Improve the safety of using medications.
- Goal 7: Reduce the risk of health care-associated infections
- Goal 8: Accurately and completely reconcile medications across the continuum of care.
- Goal 9: Reduce the risk of patient harm resulting from falls.
- Goal 13: Encourage patients' active involvement in their own care as a patient safety strategy.
- Goal 15: The organization identifies safety risks inherent in its patient population.

(Please note: Gaps in the numbering indicate that the goal is either inapplicable to the program or has been retired, typically because the requirements were integrated into the standards.)

The American Nurses Association (ANA) *Code of Ethics with Interpretive Statements* provides additional guidance for professional nursing practice. The code articulates the moral commitment to maintain the values and ethical obligations of all nurses. The ANA code and the explications for perioperative nursing provide the context within which perioperative nurses can make ethical decisions.

Quality Improvement Principles

Knowledge of the principles of quality improvement is another significant aspect of perioperative nursing care. The term "quality" is usually defined as meeting and/or exceeding the expectations and needs of the customer (Gable, et al, 1999). By definition, the focus is clearly on the customer. There are many customers in the OR, including the patients, surgeons, and staff members—all of whom have varying expectations and needs. Quality improvement is based on the following principles (Gabel, et al, 1999).

- Workers in the workplace are doing their best to perform their jobs as they understand them.

- The system in which everyone works is the primary factor in quality control.

- Management controls the system.

- Workers are in the best position to identify problems and recommend system changes, as only they can recognize what improvements are required.

- The system is comprised of the interactions among all workers, both professional and support.

- Every worker is sometimes a supplier and sometimes a customer in an interaction with coworkers.

- Clear communication between internal customers and internal suppliers is crucial to ensuring that the system works.

- Trade-offs of patient care responsibility are significant locations for communication problems between internal customers and internal suppliers and therefore are strategic points where quality improvement opportunities can be identified.

Nursing Research and Evidence-Based Practice

Nursing research on the effectiveness of patient care strategies to support evidence-based practice is an important element of professional nursing practice and also a key factor in the delivery of safe patient care. Access to and appropriate use of evidence-based data are crucial considerations in the provision of quality patient care, as optimal health care outcomes can only be achieved when the best scientific evidence is fully incorporated into clinical practices (Delbanco, 2005).

Clinical Privileges

Professional registered nurses work closely as a cohesive team with surgeons, anesthesia care providers, and a variety of specialized technical and support personnel. Each of these groups has distinctly different educational preparation, scope of practice, and professional responsibility. While most perioperative nurses are employed by the health care facility in which they work, there may be situations in which the nurse is hired as an independent contractor. In these cases, the nurse must apply for clinical privileges.

Clinical privileges involve threshold criteria that outline the training, experience, and certification an applicant must demonstrate in order to be granted core and specialty privileges in a medical or nursing specialty. A clinical privilege is a specific grant or permission by the institution for an individual practitioner to perform diagnostic or therapeutic procedures or other patient care services within well-defined limits (Kristeller, 1995). Delineation of clinical privileges is the process whereby the medical staff evaluates and recommends that an individual practitioner be allowed to provide specific patient care services in a health care facility (Kristeller, 1995). Privilege delineation is an institutional governing board function that bases the clinical privileges granted to each member on their demonstrated ability to perform, thereby ensuring patient safety and promoting quality patient care. Furthermore, some institutions are integrating the methodologies of clinical practice improvement and evidence-based practice to enable clinicians to routinely implement "best practices" in clinical care.

Performing Nursing Interventions

Anatomy and Physiology/Surgical Procedure

Because surgical procedures are classified according to their related anatomic structure or physical system, knowledge of anatomy and physiology is critical for perioperative nurses, regardless of their role in the procedure. The location and anatomical structures of the body relate to all phases of a surgical or invasive procedure. Knowledge of normal physiologic function is also essential to understanding alterations in function caused by anesthetic agents, other drugs, or the surgical intervention. Perioperative nurses should continually assess their knowledge of anatomy and physiology and its correlation to the surgical procedure being performed.

Environmental Factors

One of the perioperative nurse's greatest responsibilities as the patient's advocate is maintaining the best possible environment for surgical intervention. Two important environmental factors in the OR that must be controlled in order to accomplish this are ventilation and traffic.

Airborne microbial contamination is always a concern in the OR. An effective ventilation system is needed to minimize airborne contamination. The current requirement is a minimum of 15 total air exchanges per hour, with the equivalent of a minimum of three replacements being of fresh or outside air (Fogg, 2003). The ambient room air may need to be modified with an air conditioning system to maintain the temperature at a range of 20° to 23° C (68° to 73° F) and the humidity level of 30% to 60% (Fogg, 2003). Maintaining this humidity level helps reduce static electricity and bacterial growth.

Effective control of traffic in the OR suite protects patients, staff, supplies, and equipment from potential sources of contamination. The OR suite should be segregated from the health care facility's mainstream traffic. Traffic also should be controlled within the OR suite.

According to the AORN Recommended Practices for Traffic Patterns in the Perioperative Practice Setting, the OR suite should be divided into three areas:

- unrestricted—includes the central control point; street clothes are permitted;
- semirestricted—includes the peripheral support areas; surgical attire and head/facial hair covering are required; and
- restricted—includes the operating rooms, procedure rooms, and the clean core area; surgical attire and hair coverings are required; masks are required in the presence of open sterile supplies or scrubbed personnel.

The perioperative nurse is responsible for monitoring and managing the perioperative environment for temperature and humidity, as well as traffic patterns, personnel movements, and noise. The perioperative nurse also coordinates emergency response supplies and equipment within the sterile field, the OR environment, and the overall perioperative environment as the situation dictates.

Pharmacology and Anesthetic Agents

Pharmacology is the science that draws on information from several fields, including chemistry, anatomy, physiology, psychology, and microbiology. Because perioperative nurses are knowledgeable about these disciplines, they should maintain a good working knowledge of the pharmacologic agents most commonly used in a patient's surgical experience. Pharmacologic agents used in the perioperative setting include those that are administered via inhalation, parenterally, or topically. With all medications, the nurse must adhere to the five "Rs" of medication delivery—the right patient, medication, dose, route, and time. The nurse also must know the:

- patient's allergies;
- proper reconstitution and preparation procedures, using the manufacturer's recommendations and/or institutional policies and procedures; and
- proper dosage, routes of administration, and possible complications and side effects of every drug administered.

Facility policy should delineate the process that perioperative nurses must follow for safe medication administration. All policies and procedures should be current and based on the latest literature findings. In addition, the state nurse practice act outlines the scope of nursing practice with regard to medication administration.

Sedative/hypnotics drugs depress the central nervous system (CNS) and are often administered for premedication, moderate sedation, and supplementation of anesthesia. CNS depression is more generalized with some of these agents than with others. The mildest form of CNS depression is sedation, which diminishes physical and mental responses at lower dosages of certain CNS depressant drugs, but does not affect consciousness. Increasing the dose can produce a hypnotic affect, or a form of "natural" sleep.

Anesthetic agents are classified as either general or local. General anesthetics depress the CNS, alleviate pain, and cause loss of consciousness. Local anesthetics are agents that stop axonal conduction by blocking sodium channels in the axonal membrane. An action potential requires the movement of sodium ions from outside the axon to the inside. This influx takes place through specialized sodium channels. By blocking axonal sodium channels, local anesthetics stop sodium entry, thereby preventing conduction. Conduction is blocked only in the neurons located near the administration site. Compared to general anesthetics, the main advantage of local anesthetics is that pain can be suppressed without causing the generalized depression of the entire nervous system. Therefore, local anesthetics allow the performance of selected medical and surgical interventions with less risk than that associated with general anesthesia.

Anesthetic Interventions

Perioperative nurses also should be aware of nursing implications of anesthetic interventions. As part of the initial nursing assessment, the patient's American Society of Anesthesiology (ASA) classification, which is used to determine risk factors based on the patient's current physical/health status, should be used as a guide to help the nurse anticipate potential adverse events that may occur as a result of anesthetic intervention and/or the surgical procedure.

During induction and maintenance of anesthesia, the perioperative nurse should be aware of the potential patient responses and be prepared to intervene appropriately. For example, during induction, the patient's hearing becomes intensified. The perioperative nurse should reduce extraneous noise by closing the OR doors and reducing talking and unnecessary movement in the room. In addition, he or she should remain at the head of the OR bed to provide emotional support to the patient and assist the anesthesia care provider as needed with intubation and providing cricoid pressure. Throughout the patient's surgical experience, the perioperative nurse should remain alert to potential adverse reactions to anesthetic intervention and be prepared to assist the anesthesia care provider in all phases of general or regional anesthesia.

Principles of Positioning

Positioning is the art of moving and securing the human body into place, providing the best possible exposure of the surgical site, while allowing the least compromise in physiologic functions and mechanical stresses of the body structures and permitting access to the patient's airway, intravenous lines, and monitoring devices. The surgical patient poses special concerns for the perioperative nurse because of the inability to relate sensations of discomfort or pain, the unnatural posturing required for certain procedures, and the effects of anesthetic agents and other drugs that affect normal physiologic functions.

Patient positioning is an interdependent nursing/medical task that is performed by all professional members of the surgical team. Perioperative nurses share the responsibility and legal accountability for positioning the patient with the surgeon and anesthesia care provider. Positioning should not compromise circulatory, respiratory, integumentary, musculoskeletal, or neurological structures. Protection of these structures during positioning is a critical step in preventing untoward effects. The potential untoward effects of improper positioning include ineffective breathing patterns, impaired gas exchange, alterations in cardiac output, alterations in tactile sensory perception, impaired mobility, and impaired skin integrity.

According to the 2006 AORN Recommended Practices for Positioning the Patient in the Perioperative Practice Setting, in order to reduce the risk of injury and complications related to positioning, the perioperative nurse should:

- plan for and secure clean, working positioning devices before transfer to the OR bed as needed based on the preoperative assessment;
- actively monitor body alignment and tissue integrity; and
- evaluate the patient's body alignment and tissue integrity after positioning.

Physiologic Responses to the Surgical Experience/ Potential Complications

One of the most common complications of anesthesia and surgery that can lead to severe disability or even death is cardiac arrest. Cardiac arrest may occur because of adverse reactions to anesthesia, such as inadequate ventilation or hypoxia, or it may be due to the potential hazards of surgical intervention (e.g., blood loss, shock). In these cases, cardiopulmonary resuscitation (CPR) is often indicated and is vital to the patient's survival. It is important that the perioperative nurse remain knowledgeable of ventilation and perfusion during CPR in order to function competently in these types of emergency situations.

CPR is the immediate restoration of respiratory and circulatory functions through manual or mechanical methods, as well as the administration of appropriate pharmacologic agents, to provide ventilation and restore the heartbeat to normal sinus rhythm (Rothrock & Smith, 2003). Effective CPR results in the artificial delivery of oxygenated blood in systemic circulation at rates sufficient to preserve vital organ function until spontaneous circulation is reestablished (McGlinch & White, 2005). Circulating blood must carry oxygen supplied by pulmonary ventilation.

In these situations, ventilation may be reestablished by mouth-to-mouth breathing, or by other artificial respiration methods, such as the use of an oxygen facemask or intubation via endotracheal tube with the use of an Ambu bag or mechanical ventilator. The delivery of oxygenated blood during cardiac arrest and CPR is directly related to the effectiveness of the chest compressions (McGlinch & White, 2005). The perioperative nurse should consult the facility's CPR protocol, participate in basic life-support training and periodic practice sessions, and also be familiar with the movable CPR or crash cart, which contains all needed supplies (Rothrock & Smith, 2003).

Malignant hyperthermia syndrome (MHS) is another serious complication of general anesthesia that requires immediate action by the surgical team. MHS is a complication of general anesthesia that occurs often without preexisting symptoms or warning. In its classic form, MHS occurs during anesthesia with a volatile agent (e.g., halothane) and the depolarizing muscle relaxant succinylcholine. It produces rapid increases in temperature (rising by as much as 1° C per 5 minutes) and severe acidosis (Gronert, et al, 2005), and is a potentially fatal disorder.

MHS is a dominantly inherited trait, but it remains latent until one of the triggering agents or conditions activates the self-disseminating crisis. Malignant hyperthermia is a myopathy, characterized by an acute loss of intracellular calcium ions (Gronert, et al, 2005). The syndrome is thought to be caused by a reduction in the reuptake of calcium by the sarcoplasmic reticulum necessary for termination of muscle contraction. Therefore, muscle contraction is sustained, resulting in signs of hypermetabolism, such as acidosis, tachycardia, hypercarbia, glycolisis, hypoxemia, and heat production, and also muscle rigidity, muscle injury, and increased sympathetic nervous system activity. Hypermetabolism reflected by elevated carbon dioxide production precedes the increase in body temperature.

It is prudent for the perioperative nurse to be knowledgeable about MHS and be prepared for an MH crisis, even though it does not occur frequently. All surgical patients should be screened for a family history of MH. The perioperative nurse assesses, documents, and reports any MHS risk factors identified in the preoperative evaluation to the anesthesia care provider and other members of the surgical team. The perioperative nurse should develop a plan of care that prescribes appropriate interventions to attain the expected outcomes; the interventions should be implemented as needed. For example, in the event of an MH crisis, the perioperative nurse should assist the anesthesia care provider in turning off all anesthetic agents and replacing the anesthesia machine.

The AORN Malignant Hyperthermia Guideline provides a resource for perioperative nurses and outlines the key nursing responsibilities during an MH crisis. The following are some of the nursing interventions may be indicated.

- Recognize and report deviations in diagnostic studies.
- Use supplies and equipment within safe parameters.
- Identify physiologic status; report variances from normal (electrocardiogram, vital signs, lab values).
- Assess skin condition.
- Implement protective measures to prevent skin/tissue injury due to thermal sources.
- Administer prescribed medications and solutions (Table 1).
- Implement thermoregulation measures.
- Consult with appropriate members of the health care team to implement new treatments or change existing treatments.
- Monitor physiologic parameters: vital signs (i.e., blood pressure, pulse rate, body temperature); oximetry; capnometry; core temperature (i.e., esophageal, tympanic, axillary, rectal, bladder); urine color and output; diaphoresis; mottling of the skin.
- Administer intravenous therapy—DO NOT use lactated Ringer's solution, as it may contribute to the patient's acidosis.
- Provide postoperative instructions to patient/significant other/support person.

The MH Hotline (800-MH-HYPER [800-644-9737]) is another excellent resource for consultation in patient management. The perioperative nurse should report patients who have had acute MH episodes to the North American MH Registry of the Malignant Hyperthermia Association of the United States (MHAUS) at 412-692-5464 by means of a confidential report. The patient also can call this number to add his or her name to the registry database. (See www.mhreg.org). Patients and families can be referred to MHAUS for additional information.

A protocol for managing an MH crisis, based on the current literature, as well as an MH crisis cart—stocked with all the necessary supplies, drugs, and solutions—should be readily available in all clinical practice settings where anesthesia is administered. All members of the surgical team should be knowledgeable about the MH protocol and work together to prevent adverse outcomes from an MH crisis.

Documentation of Nursing Interventions

For all emergency situations that occur in the OR, the perioperative nurse must accurately and comprehensively document the event or crisis, the nursing interventions, and patient outcomes in the patient's medical record.

DIRECT MULTIDISCIPLINARY HEALTH CARE TEAM MEMBERS

Basic Management Techniques and Delegation

As the professional nurse in the surgical practice setting, the perioperative nurse must demonstrate basic management techniques, including delegation of duties. The practice of nursing involves critical thinking and decision-making skills. These skills take on greater significance in an emergency situation. Management, or the ability to get things done, is achieved through the use of human, physical, and technical resources. The management process consists of four separate, but integrated functions: planning, organizing, directing, and controlling the resources in the surgical practice environment (Sword, 1996).

During an emergency situation, as well as within the course of patient care, the perioperative nurse may delegate certain nursing interventions, as outlined by the state nurse practice act's legal definition of nursing. Delegation is defined as the transferring, to a competent person, the authority to perform a selected nursing task in a selected situation according to the five rights of delegation (Rothrock, 2003):

- right task,
- right circumstances,
- right person,
- right communication and direction, and
- right supervision and evaluation.

Reporting Techniques to Multidisciplinary Health Care Providers

Accurate communication of the patient's status during an emergency situation is crucial. This is especially important during the transfer of care to another health care professional in either the postanesthesia care unit (PACU) or intensive care unit (ICU). Communication of verbal orders, critical lab values, the patient's medical condition, allergies, current medications, and the presence of implants/implantable devices is vital to continuity of care and the promotion of positive outcomes.

It is important for the perioperative nurse to be aware of barriers to effective communication. The basic skills required for communication are questioning, listening, explaining, and reflecting (Maguire, 2002). Barriers to effective communication are divided into two groups: physical and emotional. Physical barriers include speech or hearing difficulties, a noisy environment, poor sight, and poor cognitive skills. Examples of emotional barriers are prejudice, perceptions, fear, aggression, or threat. Strategies to reduce these barriers include (Maguire, 2002):

- planning—structure the explanation and organizing the facts in a logical sequence;
- presentation—keep the explanations as brief as possible; and
- feedback—obtain feedback to ensure the message is understood.

TABLE 1

Medications and Solutions for Treating Malignant Hyperthermia

DANTROLENE SODIUM:

- Currently, dantrolene sodium is the only known drug that treats MH. It impairs calcium-dependent muscle contraction and controls the hypermetabolism manifestations associated with MH.
- Dantrolene should be mixed with sterile water for injection (without a bacteriostatic agent; 60 mL per 20 mg ampule) and shaken vigorously.
- Rapidly administer intravenous (IV) dantrolene sodium 2-3 mg/kg initial bolus.

SODIUM BICARBONATE:

- Used to correct metabolic acidosis (as indicated by blood gas analysis)
- Initial dose of 1-2 mEq/kg - repeat as indicated

GLUCOSE AND INSULIN:

- Used to treat hyperkalemia—give either:
  - 10 units regular insulin in 50 mL 50% glucose titrated to potassium level or
  - 0.15 u/kg regular insulin in 1 cc/kg 50% glucose

CALCIUM CHLORIDE:

- 2-5 mg/kg to treat hyperkalemia

ANTI-ARRHYTHMIC AGENTS:

- Used if dysrhythmias persist after treatment of acidosis and hyperkalemia

AVOID SOLUTIONS CONTAINING POTASSIUM

Safeguard Patients and the Health Care Team From Environmental Hazards and Disasters

Patient Rights and Responsibilities

Patients have rights, as well as responsibilities, regarding their health and the health care services they receive. On March 26, 1997, then President Clinton appointed an Advisory Commission on Consumer Protection and Quality in the Health Care Industry. The Commission issued its final report in March 1998. As part of its work, the Commission also issued a Consumer Bill of Rights and Responsibilities, which was intended to serve as a blueprint for improvement of systems and procedures that aim to protect consumers and ensure quality of care. The Patients' Bill of Rights is as follows (Health Care Quality: Patient Rights and Responsibilities):

- **Information disclosure**—The patient has the right to receive accurate and easily understood information about their health plan, health care professionals, and health care facilities. If the patient speaks another language, has a physical or mental disability, or doesn't understand something, assistance will be provided so he or she can make informed health care decisions.

- **Choice of providers and plans**—The patient has the right to a choice of health care providers that is sufficient to provide access to appropriate high-quality health care.

- **Access to emergency services**—If the patient has severe pain, an injury, or sudden illness that convinces him or her that his or her health is in serious jeopardy, the patient has the right to receive screening and stabilization emergency services whenever and wherever needed, without prior authorization or financial penalty.

- **Participation in treatment decisions**—The patient has the right to know all treatment options and to participate in decisions about care. Parents, guardians, family members, or other designated individuals can represent the patient if he or she cannot make decisions.

- **Respect and nondiscrimination**—The patient has a right to considerate, respectful, and nondiscriminatory care from physicians, health plan representatives, and other health care providers.

- **Confidentiality of health information**—The patient has the right to talk in confidence with health care providers and to have his or her health care information protected. The patient also has the right to review and copy his or her own medical record and request that the physician amend the record if it is not accurate, relevant, or complete.

- **Complaints and appeals**—The patient has the right to a fair, fast, and objective review of any complaint he or she has against the health plan, physicians, hospitals, or other health care personnel. This includes complaints about waiting times, operating hours, the conduct of health care personnel, and the adequacy of health care facilities.

The perioperative nurse must remain aware of the patient's rights and responsibilities and take appropriate actions to protect them beginning at the time of admission and continuing throughout the patient's surgical experience.

Principles of Patient Safety

Patient safety has gained renewed focus over the past several years. The National Patient Safety Foundation's (NPSF) National Agenda for Research outlined three defining characteristics of patient safety (NPSF, 2000).

- Patient safety is primarily concerned with the avoidance, prevention, and amelioration of adverse outcomes or injuries resulting from the processes of health care itself. It should be directed to all events that are described as errors, deviations, and accidents.

- Safety transpires from the interaction of the health care system components; that is, safety does not exist only within a person, department, or device. Safety improvements are dependent upon learning how safety emerges from the interactions of the components.

- Patient safety is related to "quality of care," but the two terms are not synonymous; safety is a significant subset of quality.

The NPSF has also proposed a strategy to improve patient safety through reporting (NPSF Roundtable, 2000). The major aspects of this strategy include the following.

- Patients should be informed if they have been injured while receiving care.

- Reporting on the implementation of safety practices by health care institutions should be established and made public.

- Confidential reporting to a non-regulatory national entity should be the principal vehicle to gather information on adverse events and near misses and promote learning about them.

- Existing state mandatory reporting systems should

focus on significant licensing violations.

- A National Center for Patient Safety should be established to conduct/coordinate research in this area.

Health care facilities are urged to develop policies and procedures, based on the current literature, related to creating a patient safety culture. According to the Agency for Healthcare Research and Quality (AHRQ), the term "safety culture" refers to a commitment to safety that permeates all levels of an organization, from frontline personnel to executive management. Several features describe a culture of safety, such as (Pizzi, Goldfarb, Nash, 2001):

- acknowledgment of the high-risk, error-prone nature of an organization's activities;
- a blame-free environment in which individuals are able to report errors or close calls without fear of reprimand or punishment;
- an expectation of collaboration across ranks to seek solutions to vulnerabilities; and
- a willingness on the part of the organization to direct resources for addressing safety concerns.

The AORN Guidance Statement: Creating a Patient Safety Culture provides a framework that perioperative nurses can use to foster a patient-focused safety culture and assist in the development of policies and procedures, based on current literature, that will support this culture (AORN, 2006).

Ergonomics and Body Mechanics

The health care facility, including the perioperative practice setting, presents a variety of ergonomic-based opportunities for creating a safer, healthier environment for the staff as well as the patients. According to OSHA, ergonomics is the science of fitting the job to the worker. When there is a mismatch between the physical requirements of the job and the physical capacity of the worker, work-related musculoskeletal disorders can occur. Ergonomics also involves the practice of designing equipment and work tasks to conform to the capability of the worker, thereby providing a means for adjusting the work environment and work practices to prevent injuries before they occur.

Ergonomic stressors can be classified as dynamic or static. Dynamic tasks are those in which movement is involved. They fall into several major categories, including lateral transfers of patients, lifting and handling of patients, and movement of equipment. However, the most common and perhaps the most considerable ergonomic issue in the OR relates to static postures, or those in which the same position is held for extended time periods. Duties that require a static posture in the OR include (Owen, 2000):

- continuously standing in one position during lengthy surgical procedures;
- holding a retractor for long periods; and
- supporting a patient's extremity.

Health care facilities have been identified by OSHA as environments where ergonomic stressors exist. The *Perioperative Nursing Data Set* (PNDS) provides pertinent information when looking at potential solutions to ergonomic hazards, such as "08: Patient verbalizes comfort related to transfer/transport activities." The perioperative nurse should remain aware of the ergonomic stressors within the surgical environment and take appropriate measures to prevent injuries to both patients and staff members.

Environmental Hazards, Disasters/Terrorism/ Preparedness and Response

The perioperative nurse must be prepared for other types of emergency situations that may occur in the surgical practice setting. These situations include environmental hazards, such as fires and the presence of toxic fumes, as well as natural disasters and terrorism.

Fires:
While a fire in the OR is a rare occurrence, it can be devastating in its consequences to both patients and staff. A fire occurs when the three elements that support combustion are present: an ignition source, a fuel source, and an oxidizer; collectively these are referred to as the "fire triangle." An ignition source is anything that produces heat or sparking. Some of the most common ignition sources in the OR are the electrosurgical unit (ESU), lasers, and fiberoptic equipment. Almost anything in the OR can serve as a fuel source (e.g., patient gowns, surgical attire and other protective apparel, surgical drapes and towels, dressing materials). The principal oxidizers in the OR are oxygen and nitrous oxide. Fire safety initiatives are focused on preventing the convergence of these three elements.

The best defense against a fire in the OR is a knowledgeable and prepared perioperative nurse; education and training are paramount. The perioperative nurse must know the facility's fire safety plan that addresses risk reduction strategies, fire-fighting and evacuation procedures, and the responsibilities of each member of the surgical team. The AORN Guidance Statement: Fire Prevention in the Operating Room outlines the following ECRI recommendations for staff preparedness:

- participation in fire drills;
- training on the use of fire fighting equipment; PASS

should be reviewed to operate fire extinguishers:
  - P — Pull the pin
  - A — Aim the nozzle at the base of the fire
  - S — Squeeze the handle
  - S — Sweep the stream over the base of the fire
- knowledge of the location of the medical gas panel and electrical and ventilation systems and which personnel are allowed to shut them off;
- knowledge of how to initiate the fire alarm within the facility; and
- knowledge of the protocols to notify the local fire department.

The fire plan should include RACE as the response component:

- R — Rescue the individual involved in the fire.
- A — Alarm should be sounded as soon as possible.
- C — Confine the fire.
- E — Extinguish the fire and evacuate if necessary.

In the event of a fire, the perioperative nurse should remove any burning material from the patient and extinguish it; assist in shutting off medical gas valves, electrical and ventilation systems if indicated; and assist in transporting the patient away from the fire.

Toxic fumes:
Various chemicals are used in the perioperative practice setting, many of which are classified as irritants that can be hazardous to both patients and staff members. The AORN Recommended Practices for Safe Care through Identification of Potential Hazards in the Surgical Environment state that the potential hazards associated with the chemicals used in the surgical practice setting should be identified and safe practices for their use should be established. These chemicals include, but are not limited to:

- environmental cleaning agents;
- disinfectants and sterilants;
- skin prep, degreasing, and adhesive agents;
- chemotherapeutic agents;
- tissue preservatives; and
- polymethylmethacrylate.

With some of these agents, excessive exposure to vapors can produce eye or respiratory tract irritation. Systemic reactions to high levels of noxious vapors may include dyspnea, generalized erythroderma, drowsiness, and potentially unconsciousness.

OSHA's Hazard Communication Standard, Toxic and Hazardous Substances, outlines that all employees must be informed of the hazards associated with the chemicals that are present in their work environment. It also states that material safety data sheets (MSDS) for every potentially hazardous chemical must be readily accessible to employees in the practice setting. The perioperative nurse should read and follow the instructions provided on the MSDS for the chemicals used in the surgical environment.

Disasters/Terrorism:
Perioperative nurses and the surgical team routinely face clinical emergency situations in the various surgical practice settings. However, emergency situations encountered in health care facilities include other threats such as natural disasters and terrorism. A disaster is defined as an incident that results in multiple casualties that *overwhelm* local resources; the goal for disaster response it to maximize the number of lives saved (AHRQ, 2004). Examples of natural disasters include earthquakes, hurricanes, floods, and tidal waves. Terrorist threats, or manmade disasters, include disasters caused by chemical, biological, and radiological agents, as well as bombings.

Preparedness and response:
The perioperative care areas are vital components of a health care facility's preparedness plan (Eiland, et al, 2004). All health care facilities should have an emergency preparedness plan that includes general procedures, as well as specific responses to either natural or manmade disasters. The 2006 JCAHO Hospital Accreditation Standards for Emergency Management Planning, Emergency Management Drills, Infection Control, Disaster Privileges require that emergency preparedness plans identify the specific procedures for (Eiland, et al, 2004):

- mitigation — activities undertaken to lessen the impact and severity of a potential emergency;
- preparedness — activities undertaken to build capacity and identify resources in case of an emergency;
- response — activities designed to control the negative effects of an emergency situation; and
- recovery — actions designed to restore normal operations and essential services of the health care facility.

Perioperative preparedness is especially important as part of the overall emergency plan. The perioperative nurse must be knowledgeable about individual roles and responsibilities during an emergency, assess the inventory of supplies on hand, know the procedure for obtaining additional supplies as needed; effectively implement the charge capture system, and plan in advance for recovery and return to normal service (Eiland, et al, 2004). The perioperative nurse should be familiar with the facility's emergency preparedness plan, including the information specific to perioperative preparedness, and also participate in scheduled emergency drills.

Responsibilities Regarding Impaired Practitioners and/or Disruptive Behavior

Two other unfortunate situations that perioperative nurses may encounter are dealing with impaired colleagues or practitioners and disruptive behavior displayed by colleagues or patients or their family. Health care professionals are not immune to impairment conditions. Impairment by either chemical dependency or alcohol abuse typically results in distorted or diminished clinical judgment and/or technical skills, which negatively affects patient safety. In addition, impaired individuals often display unusual behaviors, such as (US Department of Justice, Drug Enforcement Administration):

- absenteeism without notification;
- excessive number of sick days used;
- frequent disappearances from the work site or long, unexplained absences;
- excessive amounts of time spent near a drug supply;
- unreliability in keeping appointments and meeting deadlines;
- work performance that alternates between high and low productivity and may suffer from mistakes made due to inattention, poor judgment, and bad decisions;
- confusion, memory loss, and difficulty concentrating or recalling details and instructions;
- interpersonal relations with colleagues, staff, and patients suffer;
- heavy "wastage" of drugs;
- sloppy recordkeeping;
- inappropriate prescriptions for large narcotic doses;
- insistence on personal administration of injected narcotics to patients;
- deterioration in personal appearance and hygiene;
- uncharacteristic deterioration of handwriting and charting;
- wearing long sleeved clothing when inappropriate;
- personality change: mood swings, anxiety, depression, lack of impulse control, suicidal thoughts or gestures;
- patient and staff complaints about health care provider's changing attitude/behavior; and
- increasing isolation—both personal and professional.

Disruptive or abusive behavior displayed by patients and/or families can have unfavorable effects on the quality of care they receive (Linck & Phillips, 2004). Disruptive behaviors often overshadow the patients' hospitalization and may impede the nurse's ability to care for the patient in an accurate and timely manner, resulting in ineffective nursing interventions (Linck & Phillips, 2004).

Most health care facilities have policies that address the behavioral expectations of patients, employees, and contract workers in an effort to provide a working environment that is free from disruptive behaviors, abuse (verbal or physical), sexual harassment, violence, or interference with the worker's ability to perform his or her job. These policies also outline the process for identification and resolution of disruptive behavior. These policies should be based on the latest information available in the literature. Perioperative nurses, and all health care professionals, have both a legal and ethical responsibility to uphold the law and to help protect coworkers and society from abusive practitioners.

Summary

Patients scheduled for surgery or other invasive procedures are all at risk, not only from the surgical intervention and anesthesia, but in some cases from unforeseen emergency situations. One of the perioperative nurse's most important roles is that of patient advocate. In this role, the nurse must be prepared for many types of emergency situations that may occur in the surgical practice setting. Two of the expected outcomes for the surgical patient are that he or she is free from injury and infection. Teamwork is an important aspect in achieving these outcomes, but it takes on greater significance in any type of emergency situation. The perioperative nurse is in the unique role of coordinating the team effort and assisting other team members in appropriately preparing for and responding to an emergency in the OR.

Suggested Learning Activities

- Maintain certification in basic cardiac life support (BCLS).

- Review the current AORN Patient Outcome Standards and Recommended Practices.

- Review AORN Malignant Hyperthermia Guideline.

- Review the state nurse practice act to know the legal definition and scope of nursing practice.

- Maintain current knowledge on new pharmacologic agents, anesthetic agents and techniques, as well as the perioperative nurse's role in working with the anesthesia provider.

- Research the literature for perioperative disaster articles and appropriate nursing preparation strategies and actions.

- Review facility policies and procedures for emergency situations; recommend updates as needed based on current literature findings.

Chapter 8

Management of Personnel, Services, and Materials

Sherron C. Kurtz, RN, MSA, MSN, CNOR, CNAA

The preparation for the patient by the perioperative registered nurse begins when the nurse is assigned to a case. Whether the nurse is to scrub or circulate, there are some basic preparations that must be made in order to manage the environment. This includes management of personnel, services, and materials. There are critical pieces of knowledge and skills that are required for the nurse to control the perioperative environment—to control the environment for the patient and for the staff. While the patient is in a diminished state, the perioperative registered nurse functions as the patient's advocate and speaks for the patient. Therefore, it is critical that the nurse understand all aspects of controlling the environment. The nurse must control the environment to keep the patient safe and free from injury and to ensure positive patient outcomes.

This chapter provides a review of the perioperative nurse's role in the management of personnel, services, and materials. This is based on the identified task statements and the requisite knowledge and skills needed to perform these tasks. The content of this chapter will include the following focus areas:

- overview of nursing activities to manage the environment;
- safety considerations used;
- principles of equipment inspection and management techniques;
- regulatory standards and voluntary guidelines;
- nursing research;
- patient safety;
- performing nursing documentation; and
- environmental factors and their control.

Learning Objectives

Individuals preparing for the CNOR certification examination will direct their study activities toward obtaining the knowledge and skills required to appropriately manage the environment, specifically management of personnel, services, and materials. Upon completion of this chapter, the individual should be able to:

1. Describe the role of the perioperative nurse in managing the environment of the patient in surgery.
2. Discuss safety measures taken to provide patient and staff safety.
3. List four safety concerns that the nurse manages in the operating room.
4. Describe basic management techniques used by the perioperative nurse.
5. Discuss regulatory standards and voluntary guidelines used in the surgical setting.
6. Discuss aspects of product evaluation and its significance for the surgical patient.

Overview of Nursing Practice Issues Affecting the Management of Personnel, Services, and Materials

Principles of Patient Safety

In today's environment, patient safety is a key factor. In 1999, the Institute of Medicine (IOM) published the report, "To Err is Human," which identified as many as 98,000 deaths in hospitals each year that are due to preventable medical errors (IOM, 1999). Since that time, health care providers have considered patient safety as a top priority. The Joint Commission on Accreditation of Healthcare Organizations (JCAHO) has added new standards regarding patient safety and also has initiated the National Patient Safety Goals.

The Centers for Medicare and Medicaid Services (CMS) also has initiated quality initiatives. The Hospital Quality Initiative (HQI) consists of many facets and includes several goals to improve care provided by the nation's hospitals and to provide quality information to consumers (CMS, 2006).

The Association of periOperative Registered Nurses (AORN) also has identified patient safety as a high priority. This is evidenced by the "AORN Guidance Statement: Creating a Patient Safety Culture" (AORN, 2006). AORN describes the characteristics of a culture of safety as: a reporting culture, a flexible culture, a wary culture, and a just culture (AORN, 2006). Such a culture will provide an

Task/Knowledge/Skill Statements

Anticipate the needs for and acquire equipment, supplies, and personnel

- Surgical procedure
- Principles of patient safety
- Preoperative patient preparation activities
- Principles of positioning
- Instruments, supplies, and equipment relating to surgical procedure
- Principles of equipment inspection and maintenance
- Acquisition processes for equipment, supplies, and personnel
- Basic management techniques and delegation
- Nursing research and evidence-based practice

Supervise and mentor health care team members

- Communication theories and techniques (e.g., patient/family)
- Interviewing techniques (e.g., patient/family)
- Reporting techniques to multidisciplinary health care provides (e.g., critical lab values; medical condition; medications; allergies; implants/implantable devices; hand off; read back verbal orders; communication barriers)
- Basic management techniques and delegation
- Regulatory standards and voluntary guidelines (e.g., AORN *Standards, Recommended Practices and Guidelines;* OSHA; JCAHO; ANA Code of Ethics for Nurses with Explications for Perioperative Nurses; state Nurse Practice Act)
- Responsibilities regarding impaired and/or disruptive behavior (e.g., patient/family; multidisciplinary health care team members)
- Resources for professional growth (e.g., *Perioperative Nursing Data Set* [PNDS]; computer skills)
- Nursing research and evidence-based practice

Monitor cost-containment

- Patient rights and responsibilities
- Principles of patient safety
- Preoperative patient preparation activities
- Instruments, supplies, and equipment relating to surgical procedure
- Reporting techniques to multidisciplinary health care provides (e.g., critical lab values; medical condition; medications; allergies; implants/implantable devices; hand off; read back verbal orders; communication barriers)
- Principles of product evaluation and cost containment
- Quality improvement principles
- Acquisition processes for equipment, supplies, and personnel
- Basic management techniques and delegation
- Nursing research and evidence-based practice

Participate in product evaluation

- Surgical procedure
- Principles of patient safety
- Principles of wound healing
- Principles of positioning
- Ergonomics and body mechanics (e.g., patient/equipment)
- Instruments, supplies, and equipment relating to surgical procedure
- Professional and regulatory standards (e.g., AORN *Standards, Recommended Practices, and Guidelines;* Association for the Advancement of Medical Instrumentation [AAMI])
- Selecting cleaning, packaging, sterilizing, and disinfecting methods
- Principles of product evaluation and cost containment
- Quality improvement principles
- Basic management techniques and delegation
- Regulatory standards and voluntary guidelines (e.g., AORN *Standards, Recommended Practices and Guidelines*; OSHA; JCAHO; ANA Code of Ethics for Nurses with Explications for Perioperative Nurses; state Nurse Practice Act)
- Nursing research and evidence-based practice

Monitor and document the integrity and environmental condition of implanted packages (e.g., tissue; skin; bone; temperature)

- Patient rights and responsibilities
- Legal responsibilities and implications for patient care
- Principles of patient safety
- Aseptic technique
- Principles of patients' rights
- Implants (e.g., handling; tracking; sterilization)
- Documentation of all nursing interventions
- Environmental factors (e.g., temperature; humidity; air exchange; noise)
- Principles of sterilization and disinfection
- Performing and documenting sterilization procedures
- Conducting and documenting biological monitoring
- Conducting and documenting chemical monitoring
- Quality improvement principles
- Monitoring and documenting package integrity (e.g., tissue; skin; bone; temperature)
- Nursing research and evidence-based practice

atmosphere where all health care team members are open and free to discuss safety issues and errors that affect patients. A culture of safety can be identified by the characteristics of: open honest communication; emphasis on team rather than the individual; standards and practices developed in a multidisciplinary framework; trust among staff members who are supported by one another; surgical team members whose open relationship emphasizes credibility and attentiveness; and the focus is on work flow and processes (AORN, 2006).

The perioperative nurse must be aware of specific risks in the OR. To provide patients with an environment of a culture of safety, the perioperative registered nurse (RN) must ensure that the patient is brought into a safe environment. The surgical setting is one of the most potentially hazardous of all clinical settings. Infection, hemorrhage, and wrong site surgery are among the most significant patient safety issues (AORN, 2006). The hazards of the surgical care setting care are generally divided into three classifications:

- physical—ergonomic injuries, falls, noise pollution, irradiation, electricity, and fire;
- chemical—anesthetic gases, toxic fumes from gases and liquids, cytotoxic drugs, and cleaning agents; and
- biological—the patient (as host for pathogens and microorganisms), infections, waste, sharps injuries, surgical plume, and latex sensitivity.

AORN has added two other classifications to the list—psychosocial and cultural. Psychosocial issues include long hours; mandatory overtime; demographic diversity; nursing shortage; call; trauma; burnout; abuse (verbal and physical); and violence from patients, staff, and physicians. The last classification is cultural, which includes tolerance for abuse from physicians; lack of commitment by management to adhere to an optimal workplace safety program; absence of respect from peers and other health care professionals; and absence of a code of conduct for all team members (AORN, 2006).

Perioperative settings host a variety of energy sources, such as electrical, thermal, laser, and radiologic, that can be potential safety hazards. Electrical and fire safety must be considered for all areas of surgical services. Fire safety is a significant consideration because of the use of energy sources and high concentrations of oxygen. The perioperative RN must assess the room to determine if the environment is indeed safe and that no electrical or fire hazards exist. The nurse should ensure that all equipment is in proper working order. The cords on all equipment should be checked for fraying and all equipment visually checked for proper order (AORN, 2006). The perioperative nurse must take precautions such as using laser safe endotracheal tubes and moist towels to prevent reflection when using a laser. When using an electrosurgical unit, the nurse must consider skin precautions and other safety precautions to prevent pad site burns and stray current burns.

The nurse must take precautions to protect both patients and staff from ionizing radiation. The patient's body areas should be shielded from the radiation beam. Areas of particular interest are ovaries and testes, lymphatic tissue, thyroid gland, and eyes. The three factors for staff to always remember regarding radiation exposure are time, distance, and shielding (Phillips, 2004). All radiation exposure to staff must be monitored and reported to those staff members.

There are chemical risks associated with surgical procedures. These include medications, antiseptics, cements, intravascular dyes, disinfecting solutions, and irrigations solutions (AORN, 2006). Other chemical risks include anesthetic gases, cytotoxic drugs, and toxic fumes from chemicals such as cement (Phillips, 2004).

Biologicals represent other safety hazards to patients and staff. Examples of these include bloodborne pathogens; drug resistant organisms (AORN, 2006); infectious waste; surgical plume; and latex sensitivity (Phillips. 2004). The perioperative RN must understand how to manage all of these risks as well as the appropriate safety precautions to take to protect the patient and staff.

Another safety hazard is the vast amount of equipment and devices used in the OR. Examples include powered equipment, powered instruments, defibrillators, tourniquets, electrosurgical units, and positioning devices (AORN, 2006). Specific measures must be taken to provide a safe environment for patients and staff. An example would be extra safety precautions (padding to protect the patient's skin and nerves) that should be taken when using pneumatic tourniquets.

As the patient's advocate, the perioperative RN is responsible for examining the surgical environment for potential safety hazards. He or she must understand all potential hazards and know how to prevent them from occurring, and also how to handle any complications that may occur inadvertently.

Preoperative Patient Preparation Activities

There are specific activities to be completed before the patient enters the OR. "The preoperative physical preparation is designed to help all patients overcome the stresses of anesthesia, pain, fluid and blood loss, immobilization, and tissue trauma" (Phillips, 2004). Preoperative preparation includes the following components: history and physical, laboratory tests, blood type and crossmatch (if appropriate), chest x-ray (if appropriate), electrocardiogram (if appropriate), diagnostic procedures, written instructions, informed consent, nurse interview, and anesthesia assessment. The written instructions tell the patient information such as NPO status, whether to take oral medications, remove nail polish, leave jewelry and valuables at home, and what to expect the morning of surgery. Some patients, such as orthopedic and open-heart patients, require a scrub with a bactericidal agent. The patient may complete this scrub at home the night before surgery, or a preoperative nurse might complete it the morning of surgery.

The morning of surgery, the nurse performs an assessment of the patient. The nurse reviews the medical record to be certain that all physician orders have been carried out. The nurse verifies that all lab work and other tests results are within normal limits. Should something be out of normal range, the nurse notifies the surgeon and the anesthesia care provider. Most patients have an IV catheter inserted and receive fluids so that they will not become dehydrated due to the NPO status, as well as to provide IV access during surgery. The nurse answers any questions the patient and his or her family might have and ensures that the patient is comfortable and not overly anxious.

Basic Management Techniques and Delegation

A perioperative RN must learn to manage many factors in the OR. Many facets of this management process depend on the procedure—how complicated it is; how many staff members will be present; supplies and equipment needed; special needs of the patient; as well as surgeon practice and preference. The circulating nurse is the team leader. There are some basic management skills that every nurse must practice and strive to master: communicating, listening, motivating, planning, organizing, evaluating, coaching, problem solving, and decision making (Stauder, 2006).

Interpersonal skills are critical in the OR. The nurse will often need to request that staff members change gowns or gloves due to contamination. He or she must know how to tell the scrub person or even the surgeon that they are contaminated without offending them.

Good communication skills are essential; team members must communicate effectively and succinctly. During a procedure is not the time to have a communication problem. Therefore, nurses must hone their communications skills so that they can facilitate communication within the OR suite. A big part of communication is listening. It is essential that nurses listen so that they are prepared to deliver supplies to the sterile filed and to notify the team members of issues.

All student nurses learn the value of planning, and planning is critical to a perioperative nurse. The nurse must plan every aspect of care for each patient based on the surgical procedure, the surgeon, and the special needs of the patient. The perioperative RN may delegate tasks to appropriately qualified allied health personnel, but the nurse is always responsible for the actions of those personnel. The nurse can delegate tasks, but not responsibility.

After planning, the nurse must organize aspects of care and an order in which to proceed. One cannot very well insert a Foley catheter after the patient has been prepped and draped. The nursing process teaches the nurse to evaluate all aspects of patient care and all nursing actions. Evaluation begins the moment the perioperative nurse meets the patient.

Coaching is an invaluable skill for nurses. They often must coach unlicensed assistive personnel as to an appropriate behavior and execution of tasks. Perioperative RNs work diligently to improve their problem solving skills. These skills will allow them to help the team out of many difficult situations.

Lastly, decision making cannot be emphasized enough. Nurses must learn to make decisions and to be decisive about those decisions. They should be open to suggestions from others, but should be strong in the conviction that they have made the right decision.

Surgical Procedure

Preparation by the perioperative RN begins when he or she is assigned to a case. Whether the nurse is to scrub or circulate, there are basic preparations that must be completed. The nurse must consider the type of surgery to be performed and the surgeon who is performing that surgery. The perioperative RN has the basic knowledge of the various types of surgical procedures; however, if a nurse finds himself or herself assigned to a case that they are unfamiliar with, an education session is in order. Operating rooms have resource books available that can be used to look up information about particular procedures. The internet also is a good tool to research various aspects of surgical procedures to which the nurse has been assigned. The perioperative RN must know and understand what is required of the surgical procedure in order to prepare for and assist the patient.

While the perioperative nurse has a basic knowledge of each type of surgery, including the standard instruments, supplies, and equipment, specific details can be found on each surgeon's "preference card" for that procedure. The preference card lists the surgeon's gown and glove sizes, as well as preferences for special instruments, supplies, equipment, or solutions; patient positioning; sutures; and any other specific requests. It is in the best interest of each staff member to have accurate, detailed information on the preference cards for each surgeon's specific needs for every type of procedure. This allows the surgical team to be prepared and to have all items needed for the procedure ready.

The perioperative RN assembles the supplies and equipment after reviewing the preference card in detail. Again, this may require many different types of activity. Some nurses simply need to pull a case cart, completed by someone else ahead of time, which contains all needed supplies and equipment. Other nurses will need to gather all supplies listed on the preference card. This is usually completed the day or night before surgery. It is the responsibility of the perioperative RN to determine whether the appropriate supplies and instruments are present when they are pulled ahead of time. Missing supplies or equipment can cause dangerous and unnecessary delays during surgery. Any time during a surgical procedure that a supply, piece of equipment, or instrument is not listed on the preference card or has changed, the nurse should make a note to update the preference card after the procedure. This will ensure that the staff members have accurate information for the next case.

Nursing Research and Evidence-Based Practice

Incorporating nursing research into nursing practice is a challenge for administrators, managers, and staff nurses. Nurses work in a chaotic, stressful, and demanding environment when they deliver nursing care. It is essential that nurses utilize nursing research, and thereby evidence-based practice, to improve their practices. "Evidence-based practice is reflective of scientific principles, rather than tradition, habit, or outdated information" (Luby, et al, 2006).

Utilizing evidence-based practice is not as difficult as it sounds. Nurses are encouraged to question traditional practice when they are aware of nursing research. One expert encourages nurses to utilize nursing research easily by forming a journal club with others in their unit (Luby, et al, 2006). By reading, sharing, and discussing journal articles, nurses are challenged to review their practices and determine if there are better ways (evidence-based) to care for their patients. This is a good way for nurses to stay current on the latest nursing research. By utilizing current nursing research in the practice setting, nurses effectively contribute to improved patient outcomes.

Reporting Techniques to Multidisciplinary Health Care Providers

Reporting from one health care provider to another is critical to patient safety. It has been shown that the transfer of patients from one health care provider to another is a very significant time during a patient's care. Poor communication can lead to dangerous errors, and those errors can be detrimental to patient safety.

Hand-off of patient care is addressed in the JCAHO National Patient Safety Goals (NPSGs). The 2007 NPSGs include, under Goal 2, Improve the effectiveness of communication among caregivers: "Implement a standardized approach to 'hand off' communications, including an opportunity to ask and respond to questions" (JCAHO, 2006). This communication must be interactive. Therefore, a taped report may no longer be acceptable.

Nurses are challenged to provide accurate information regarding patient care, treatments and services, current condition, and any recent or anticipated changes. This information must be accurate to meet the patient safety goals. There also should be no interruptions during the hand-offs to minimize the possibility that information fails to be conveyed or forgotten (JCAHO, 2006). Nurses are developing a number of approaches to hand-offs. All of these approaches and their specific tools focus on appropriate communication to provide optimal patient care and reduce the number of errors associated with hand-offs.

Principles of Product Evaluation and Cost Containment

To ensure patient safety, a facility must have a standardized process and method for evaluating and selecting products to be used in the perioperative setting. Each perioperative practice setting will have a policy on product evaluation and selection. According to the AORN Recommended Practices for Product Selection in Perioperative Practice Settings, nurses must first consider patient safety when evaluating and selecting medical devices and products (AORN, 2006). Further, the recommended practices state that the "goals of product standardization and value analysis are to select functional and reliable products that are safe, cost-effective, and environmentally conscious that promote quality care and avoid duplication or rapid obsolescence" (AORN, 2006).

When a nurse participates in a product evaluation, there must be objective criteria established ahead of time that will be measured to judge the success of the evaluation. When a product evaluation is requested, the nurse must ascertain that this is being initiated based on an identified need for opportunity. When the evaluation is complete, an analysis is performed. Factors such as ability to standardize, cost benefit ratio, safety, ease of use, turn over of product, and complexity of product should be used to consider purchase. Using a process of this nature will protect the facility, the staff, and ultimately the patient.

Instruments, Supplies, and Equipment Relating to Surgical Procedures

The perioperative nurse is responsible for ensuring that all instruments, supplies, equipment are available before the patient enters the OR. The nurse also must assess each item to be certain it is in appropriate working condition. Instrument wrappers are inspected to ensure there are no holes or tears in the wrappers. All sterile supply packaging is inspected for package integrity. Any package integrity that is in doubt is considered contaminated. All equipment must be verified as safe.

Supplies and instruments have become a bigger issue as more prostheses and implants are used that require the attendance of health care industry representatives in the OR. Both AORN and JCAHO have recognized this. AORN has addressed the presence of industry representatives in the OR in its position statement, "AORN Statement on the Role of the Health Care Industry Representative in the Operating Room" (AORN, 2006). Through this statement, AORN believes that, in defined conditions, health care industry representatives can provide technical assistance to the surgical team, which expedites the procedure and facilitates the desired patient outcomes (AORN, 2006). Facilities should develop policies that address the presence of industry representatives in the OR.

As part of the "Universal Protocol for Preventing Wrong Site, Wrong Procedure, Wrong Person Surgery," the nurse must now ensure that all implants are present in the room before the incision is made (JCAHO, 2006). This provides another safety step for surgical patients.

Patient Rights and Responsibilities

Many consider health care as a partnership between patients and health care providers. Part of this partnership includes the patient's rights and responsibilities. Nurses are committed to protecting patient's personal, moral, and legal rights (Rothrock, 2003). The course of action involves correctly identifying patients; safeguarding their right to privacy and their right to make choices regarding their care; and keeping all personal health information confidential. The Health Insurance Portability and Accountability Act (HIPAA) gives patients significant rights over how their personal health information is used. Today, hospitals must have administrative procedures in place to protect the privacy and confidentiality of patients (Rothrock, 2003).

Patient rights can be broken down into the following categories:

- rights related to the people caring for the patient;
- rights related to patient care;
- rights to personal privacy, dignity, and confidentiality;
- rights related to needs or questions patients have in the hospital;
- rights related to a patient's health care decision;
- rights related to compliments, concerns, and grievances;
- rights regarding complaints about the hospital or caregiver; and
- rights about patient safety.

Patients also have responsibilities to the hospital and health care providers. They are responsible for delivering effective information to the health care provider; cooperating with the health care team; and participating in a safe environment (e.g., no smoking, no alcohol, keeping noise levels to a minimum).

Quality Improvement Principles

"Quality improvement (QI) and performance improvement (PI) are specific methods of control that focus on improvement" (Peterson, 2004). Although there have been a number of different names for hospital improvement processes, they are all based on the premise that quality can be assessed, measured, and improved. Quality improvement is a management function that examines processes in order for staff nurses and nurse managers to identify process problems. After process problems are identified, teams are formed to identify solutions for these issues and problems. Quality improvement implements action designed to eliminate real or potential problems and improve patient outcomes.

Quality improvement goes back to the nursing process—assess the situation, identify the problem or issue, use multiple people to help plan a solution, find a better process to alleviate the problem, and implement change to resolve the issues. Then there must be evaluation to verify that the proper solution is in place. The function of quality improvement should be embraced and used by all perioperative nurses to improve patient care and provide more positive patient outcomes.

Anticipate the Needs For and Acquire Equipment, Supplies, and Personnel

Principles of Positioning

Before the patient is brought into the OR, the perioperative nurse should review the proposed position by using knowledge of the procedure and the surgeon's preference cards. The nurse verifies that the appropriate bed is in place and that it is functioning correctly. Proper positioning is critical because of the complications that might

occur. These complications include, but are not limited to:

- hemodynamic instability by orthostatic position,
- poor ventilation,
- peripheral nerve damage,
- tissue damage,
- ischemia,
- compartment syndrome,
- corneal abrasion,
- blindness from optic nerve ischemia,
- pressure necrosis,
- digit amputation in table bends,
- ischemic limbs from arterial occlusion, and
- venous emboli (Phillips, 2004).

The patient's position for surgery is determined by the surgical procedure to be performed, the surgeon's preferred approach, and the techniques of anesthesia administration (Phillips, 2004). Preoperatively, the nurse must assess the patient's skin condition and identify any problem areas, identify any limits of mobility, and determine if the patient has any prostheses (such as a total hip or knee). The patient's position should provide maximum exposure for the surgeon and access to intravenous (IV) lines and monitoring devices (AORN, 2006).

Patient positioning is a team function. The nurse must ensure that there are an adequate number of people to move the patient after induction. The surgeon often will guide the positioning process. There are a variety of position aids that the nurse should have in the room. These include, but are not limited to:

- support devices (e.g., foam pads, gelpads, thoracic rolls, pillows, wedges);
- pads in a variety of shapes, sizes, and material for protecting pressure points;
- securing devices (e.g., straps, belts, tape, kidney rests, vacuum pack positioning devices);
- procedure bed equipment (e.g., stirrups, footboards, headrest holders armboards); and
- specialty surgical beds, such as fracture tables (AORN, 2006).

After the patient is positioned, the perioperative nurse must verify that all bony prominences are padded; the patient's circulation is not impaired; extremities, thus peripheral nerves, are in appropriate alignment and supported; body weight is evenly distributed; and that all body parts are in proper alignment. This will help prevent injuries caused by positioning.

Principles of Equipment Inspection and Maintenance

All equipment must be verified as safe; there must be a current safety check sticker from the biomedical engineering department. The nurse visually inspects equipment for obvious physical damage (e.g., frayed cords, missing pieces). Any time a piece of equipment looks or acts suspicious, the nurse should have biomedical engineering assess the equipment. If a piece of equipment fails to work properly, the nurse must remove the equipment from the OR, label it with a description of the problem, and secure it so that biomedical engineering can check it. Broken or suspicious equipment must not be used on any patient until biomedical engineering has ensured that it is in proper working order.

Supervise and Mentor Health Care Team Members

Communication Theories and Techniques

Communication in nursing is of vital importance; the goal of communication is to exchange information. The nurse must be aware of basic communication techniques to communicate effectively with patient and their families. The nurse will ask the patient many questions, and open-ended questions will solicit more in-depth responses. These questions require patients to reflect and to describe their health history and physical status in greater detail, rather than give a simple one-word answer. They can also solicit problems that the nurse should be aware of.

Effective communication among caregivers regarding a patient is critical to patient safety. JCAHO has deemed it critical to patient safety as evidenced by the 2007 National Patient Safety Goals. Goal 2 states "Improve the effectiveness of communication among caregivers" (JCAHO, 2006). Ineffective communication has been shown to be a root cause of a number of sentinel events. Effective communication must be timely, accurate, unambiguous, and understood by the recipient. Good communication reduces errors and improves patient safety (JCAHO, 2006).

Interviewing Techniques

Active listening skills are effective in delving deeper into the patient's comments. The nurse can encourage the patient to continue by comments such as "yes" or "go on." By restating, the nurse can ensure that he or she understands the patient's communication. Silence will encourage the patient to talk more, often revealing a better picture of his or her health.

When conducting a patient interview, the perioperative nurse must pay particular attention to the patient's body language. A patient can deny pain, but give strong evidence of denied pain by grimacing, positioning, or muscle tension. In such situations, the nurse should attempt to solicit an accurate picture of the patient's pain. As previously stated, a much greater wealth of information will be obtained through asking open-ended questions. This requires the patient to comment and to give greater detail than simple one-word answers.

Regulatory Standards and Voluntary Guidelines

Today, perioperative nurses practice under a plethora of regulatory and professional voluntary guidelines. The perioperative nurse should have a keen awareness of relevant professional practice guidelines. These regulations and guidelines support perioperative practice by leading nurses to safe and effective professional practice. There are a number of federal and state regulations that govern practice and determine if a health care facility is allowed to remain open to care for patients. They also determine whether they can receive payment from government payers such as CMS for Medicare and Medicaid patients and Tricare for military personnel and dependents.

The Occupation Safety and Health Act of 1970 created the Occupational Safety and Health Administration (OSHA) as part of the U.S. Department of Labor. OSHA is responsible for developing and enforcing workplace safety and health regulations that, if followed, ensure a safe environment for workers. OSHA describes its mission as "to assure the safety and health of America's workers by setting and enforcing standards; providing training, outreach, and education; establishing partnerships; and encouraging continual improvement in workplace safety and health" (OSHA, 2006). Facilities must adhere to OSHA regulations or face significant fines. OSHA guidelines cover many aspects of practice to provide workplace safety. Aspects of perioperative practice governed by OSHA include blood and body fluid exposure; exposure to chemicals (e.g., anesthesia gases, disinfectants, sterilization chemicals); ergonomic issues, and exposure to physical hazards (e.g., fires, electrical, radiation, lasers).

The Centers for Disease Control and Prevention (CDC) is part of the U.S. Department of Health and Human Services (HHS). The CDC strives to protect the health and safety of people in the United States and throughout the world. They provide reliable health information and improve health through strong partnerships. Their mission is "to promote health and quality of life by preventing and controlling disease, injury, and disability" (CDC, 2006). The CDC seeks to accomplish its mission by working with partners throughout the nation and the world to: monitor health; detect and investigate health problems; conduct research to enhance prevention; develop and advocate sound public health policies; implement prevention strategies; promote healthy behaviors; foster safe and healthful environments; and provide leadership and training (CDC, 2006).

Much of the CDC information that relates to perioperative nursing practice comes from the Healthcare Infection Control Practices Advisory Committee (HICPAC). HICPAC is a federal advisory committee that provides advice and guidance to the CDC regarding the practice of health care infection control and strategies for surveillance, prevention, and control of health care associated infections in health care facilities. The committee issues recommendations for preventing and controlling health care associated infections in the form of guidelines, resolutions, and informal communications (HICPAC, 2006). The Guideline for Prevention of Surgical Site Infection, published in 1999, presents the CDC's recommendations for the prevention of surgical site infections (SSI), previously called surgical wound infections. These guidelines are a basis for many practices concerning surgical patients, surgical team members, and the physical environment of the OR. These guidelines advise health care professionals regarding many issues affecting surgical patients including: hand antisepsis, the OR environment, asepsis, hair removal, and skin preparation. Many of AORN's recommended practices are based on these CDC guidelines.

The National Institute for Occupational Safety and Health (NIOSH) is the federal agency responsible for conducting research and making recommendations for the prevention of work-related injury and illness. NIOSH is part of the CDC, which is part of HHS. NIOSH helps ensure safe and healthful working conditions for working men and women by providing research, information, education, and training in the field of occupational safety and health. NIOSH objectives are: to conduct research to reduce work-related illnesses and injuries; promote safe and healthy workplaces through interventions, recommendations, and capacity building; and enhance global workplace safety and health through organizations and international collaborations (NIOSH, 2006).

The JCAHO's mission is "to continuously improve the safety and quality of care provided to the public through the provision of health care accreditation and related services that support performance improvement in health care" (JCAHO, 2006). JCAHO is the body that accredits hospitals through surveys that ensure that safe effective patient care is being provided by assessing a hospital's compliance with their standards. These standards cover many aspects of perioperative nursing, such as the Universal Protocol for Preventing Wrong Site, Wrong Procedure, Wrong Person Surgery (JCAHO, 2006). The JCAHO has led us to many of the ideas that we consider in our practice today. A few examples are competency standards, documentation of sterilization and disinfection, and performance improvement.

One of the newest and most significant contributions of JCAHO is the National Patient Safety Goals. The purpose of the Joint Commission's National Patient Safety Goals (NPSG) is to promote specific improvements in patient safety. The goals are created to address problematic areas in health care often focusing on previous sentinel events. They describe evidence and expert-based solutions to these identified problems. After the goal has been on the list for some time and hospitals have demonstrated compliance, the goal transitions to a standard. The standard for prevention of wrong site, wrong surgery, wrong patient surgery was once a NPSG and is now a standard. The standard for reducing the risk of surgical fires also was once a NPSG.

The American Nurses Association (ANA), the professional association for all registered nurses, publishes the ANA *Code of Ethics for Nurses with Interpretive Statements.* The Code of Ethics is a succinct statement of the ethical obligations and duties of every professional nurse. It is the profession's nonnegotiable ethical standard. And it is an expression of nursing's own understanding of its commitment to society (AORN, 2006). AORN offers an interpretation of this code of ethics for the perioperative practice setting (AORN. 2006). This provides a context for perioperative nursing practice.

Responsibilities Regarding Impaired and/or Disruptive Behavior

Every nurse has a responsibility regarding impaired professionals. The problem of health care professionals impaired by alcohol, drugs, and mental health problems was often ignored until late in the last century. Professionals become impaired as a result of chemical substance abuse that includes alcohol, drugs, or narcotics. Today, chemical dependency is seen as a controllable disease. The impaired professional presents a serious danger to patients and other health care professionals.

Every nurse must be alert to indicators of chemical dependency, such as:

- absenteeism,
- "on-the-job" absenteeism,
- difficulty in concentration,
- inconsistent work patterns,
- physical/emotional problems,
- decreasing job efficiency,
- poor relationships on the job,
- medication-centered problems, and
- personal life interference with job. (Georgia Nurses Association, 2006).

The perioperative nurse must alert the manager if any health care professional exhibits any symptoms of impairment. There are programs among most state boards of nursing and medicine that will assist professionals with treatment and follow-up. The nurse must not believe that he or she is doing the impaired professional a favor by not reporting them. Reporting the professional is the only way he or she will receive the needed assistance. Health care professionals in the perioperative setting are at greater risk for chemical dependency due to the frequency of handling and sometimes ease of obtaining controlled substances.

Another problem that affects professionals and patients in hospitals is disruptive behavior. Historically, this has been thought of as a physician problem; today, however, we recognize that nurses also may exhibit disruptive behavior. This has been and may continue to be a significant problem in the OR where professionals work in a highly stressful and challenging environment. For many years, bad behavior was ignored in surgery because of the stressful nature of surgery. Disruptive behavior jeopardizes patient care, compromises teamwork, and erodes morale. Staff members and administrators must be educated to recognize and address disruptive behavior in a professional manner. Nurses must insist on a zero tolerance of disruptive behavior.

While it is easy for nurses to recognize physician disruptive behavior, they seldom recognize nurse-to-nurse or nurse-to-technologist disruptive behavior, know as horizontal violence. This also could be called interpersonal conflict or bullying. Horizontal violence may be even more disturbing than disruptive physician behavior because it comes from a peer (Leiper, 2005). Nurse-to-nurse hostility can take many forms, including:

- criticizing,
- blaming,
- scapegoating,
- undermining,
- infighting,
- sabotaging, and
- bickering (Leiper, 2005).

This violence also includes nurses being rude, verbally abusive, humiliating, or unjustly critical. Researchers categorize aggression as active or passive. Active aggression ranges from criticizing or even screaming at another nurse to physical assault. Passive aggression is less direct and more subtle. It may include talking behind a colleague's back, withholding information needed for job completion, and ignoring one another (Leiper, 2005).

Nurses must take a stand. They must not allow horizontal violence to continue. Nurses can identify and report this violence. Management is required to deal with this type of behavior once it is reported. One of the best ways to deal with this behavior is peer to peer. If a nurse witnesses this type of behavior, it is appropriate to say something about the behavior. Identify the behavior and tell the person talking that this is horizontal violence, is detrimental to the individual and the team, and should stop. This is a true challenge, but is the appropriate step for a professional nurse to take. If all staff members will challenge horizontal violence in this manner, it will stop.

Resources for Professional Growth

Perioperative nurses must continually assess their knowledge and skill level. This assessment will allow nurses to identify areas for professional growth and development. After identifying those areas that have opportunity for growth, nurses should seek out appropriate resources. Nurses can grow through pursuit of advanced nursing degrees.

One significant method for growth and development is found through professional associations. Nurses gain much from their national nursing associations, state nursing associations, and specialty associations. There nurses can find mentors and other colleagues to share ideas and opportunities. Volunteering and becoming involved in professional associations elevates a nurse's practice through gaining knowledge and awareness of regulatory and legal aspects of professional nursing, the governance aspects of the organization, and seminars and educational offerings provided by the association.

Certification also is an area for professional growth. Certification demonstrates a nurse's commitment to professional growth and practice. Involvement in the development of the certification process challenges a nurse and offers him or her significant opportunity for professional development.

Monitor Cost Containment

Acquisition Processes for Equipment, Supplies, and Personnel

Perioperative nurses must be aware of how to obtain supplies, equipment, and additional personnel when needed. Facilities have processes in place for supply acquisition. Nurses need to understand the required paperwork to use and whom to call if they have an emergency. This will vary from facility to facility, and much depends on the size of the institution. Is it a 30-suite operating room or a 2-room ambulatory surgery center? There is a big difference. The nurse in a large facility may simply have to make a phone call to have supplies delivered. The nurse in the ambulatory setting might only have to make a phone call as well, but the challenge may be knowing who to call. Surgical service leadership has these policies defined, and nurses must understand the policies and know how to implement them.

The perioperative nurse is the person who will call for additional human resources, such as medical imaging personnel or personnel for technical assistance. The nurse must constantly be aware of what the surgeon is doing and where the surgeon is in the procedure so that he or she can arrange for all additional supplies and equipment, as well as human resources to be present at the right time. The nurse must use her critical thinking skills to help the team acquire needed items. By doing this, the perioperative nurse can provide the patient with a better chance for a positive outcome by being prepared and reducing any wait time.

Participate in Product Evaluation

Principles of Wound Healing

After a surgical procedure, the normal barrier function of skin is destroyed by the surgical incision. In an uncompromised patient, wounds heal spontaneously and without complications. A closed wound, such as an incision, heals by primary intention and has accurately approximated edges (Gruendemann & Mangum, 2001). Key elements of primary closure or first intention include: no tissue loss; well-approximated edges with suture, wound sealant, or wound-closure strips; minimal or no postoperative swelling; no serious discharge or local infection; no separation of would edges; and minimal scar formation (Phillips, 2004).

Basically, an incision begins a series of events that form clots, and the healing continues for about 21 days (Gruendemann & Mangum, 2001). There are three distinct phases of wound healing: lag phase of acute inflammatory response, healing or proliferative of fibroplasias, and maturation (Phillips, 2004). The maturation phase of healing begins after the 21 days and may continue for up to a year. Collagen forms and fibers begin to criss-cross and build a strong network so that the tensile strength of the wound is increased. Scaring occurs and resolves (Gruendemann & Mangum, 2001).

Secondary wound healing results when wound closure occurs through granulation, re-epithelialization, and contraction, rather than by closing the wound with sutures (Gruendemann & Mangum, 2001). The wound will heal spontaneously. There are a number of considerations with this type of healing.

- Infection, excessive trauma, loss of tissue, or poorly approximated edges are common.
- Inflammatory response is exaggerated.
- The wound is left open and allowed to heal from the inside to the outside tissues.
- Healing is delayed, and the wound may need a skin graft.

- Healing may produce a weak union that might lead to an incisional hernia later on.
- The risk of infection is proportionate to the amount of necrotic tissue present in the wound.
- Scar formation is excessive.
- Contraction of skins is pronounced (Phillips, 2004).

Third intention, or delayed primary closure, occurs when the surgeon delays wound closure for the purpose of walling off an area of gross infection or where extensive tissue has been removed. The wound is usually closed 4 to 6 days postoperatively. The following are considerations for healing by third intention.

- The wound is cleaned and debrided.
- The wound is packed with moist gauze to promote drainage and granulation.
- Antibiotic therapy is initiated.
- The wound may be an old traumatic or septic wound.
- Deep sutures should be avoided.
- Two clean surfaces of granulation are brought together for later closure.
- A deeper and wider scar usually exists (Phillips, 2004).

Ergonomics and Body Mechanics

Back injury is a leading cause of missed time from work for nurses. It is reported that each year 12% of registered nurses leave nursing because of back injury, and more than 53% complain of chronic back pain (AORN Online, 2006). Good body mechanics and use of ergonomic principles protect OR employees and thereby influence good practice. Personnel should be educated and supervised in the use of equipment to prevent injury. Standing for long periods of time is a common cause of low back pain—particularly if standing in an awkward position (AORN Online, 2006).

Shoes should be considered for safety and comfort. Canvas or leather shoes with ties are best. The OR bed should be adjusted to a reasonable height so as not to create a strain for scrubbed personnel. Good body posture is a valuable tool in assisting with good back health. First assistants can develop carpal tunnel by holding retractors. There are a number of principles of body mechanics that should be considered. These principles are considered not only for staff while delivering patient care, but also when new products are being evaluated. Principles of body mechanics are important to all staff members.

- Keep the body close to the person or equipment to be moved.
- Lift with the large muscles of your legs and abdominal muscles—not the back.
- Bend the knees to get body weight under the load.
- Lift with a slow, even motion.
- Push—do not pull—stretchers, tables, or heavy equipment.
- Use large body muscles to maneuver the base of heavy equipment.
- If standing for a prolonged period of time, stand in a wide stance.
- Distribute weight evenly on both legs.
- Sit with the back straight.
- Align the head and neck and bend forward from the hips.
- Change positions, stretch, or walk out of the rooms at intervals.
- Pivot the entire body to avoid twisting at the waist.
- Avoid overhead reaching (Phillips, 2004).

There are many devices that can assist the nurse with body mechanics. Facilities should arrange for devices that assist the nurse in moving the patient. Many hospitals now have a "no-lift" policy. Nurses should be involved in the selection of lifting aides and products. Nurses also should be involved in the selection of all products and equipment so that they can consider any positions or movements that are detrimental to good body mechanics.

Monitor and Document the Integrity and Environmental Condition of Implanted Packages

Legal Responsibilities and Implications for Patient Care

In 2004, U. S. Food and Drug Administration (FDA) published its rule, "Current Good Tissue Practice for Human Cell, Tissue, and Cellular and Tissue-Based Product Establishments; Inspection and Enforcement." This rule requires facilities that recover, process, store, label, package, or distribute tissue to follow current good tissue practice requirements. This rule also allows the FDA to inspect facilities and to enforce the regulations (FDA, 2006).

The nurse has a legal responsibility to patients regarding integrity and environmental conditions related to the packaging of implanted skin, tissue, or bone. Most hospitals do not procure, process, or preserve tissue; however, they do store tissue prior to implantation. These hospitals are required to have defined oversight of tissue with authority and accountability for all activities (AORN, 2006). Hospitals are required to maintain records of receipt, records of storage, and records of dispersement on all implanted tissue (FDA, 2006). A hospital must be able to track a piece of tissue, should it be recalled.

These requirements are all good practice for surgical patients, but they also fulfill a legal responsibility to the patient. Negligence is defined as failure to use the care or skills that any caregiver in the same or similar situation would be expected to use. All tissue for implantation must be maintained properly. If a nurse implants tissue that has not been stored properly and there is a problem with the patient later, there could be malpractice liability.

Malpractice is, among other things, any unreasonable lack of skill or judgment. The four "Ds" of malpractice are described as: duty to deliver a standard of care; deviation from that duty by omission or commission; direct causation of damage because of a deviation; and damages to a patient caused by said deviation from the standard of care (Phillips, 2004). Consider applying that to tissue; for example, a patient has a problem after a tissue implantation. If the facility cannot produce records that describe appropriate care of that tissue, such as temperature logs, there may well be a malpractice case and the hospital is liable for any patient adverse response.

Aseptic Technique

Aseptic technique is the method used to prevent microbial contamination in the environment; it is used to protect patients and health care providers. Aseptic practices are used preoperatively, intraoperatively, and postoperatively to minimize wound contamination and reduce patient risk for surgical site infection (AORN, 2006). There are several key practices used to provide aseptic technique:

- Scrubbed persons should function within a sterile field.
- Sterile drapes should be used to establish a sterile field.
- Items in the sterile field must be sterile.
- Items are either sterile or unsterile.
- A sterile field should be maintained and monitored constantly (AORN, 2006).

The perioperative nurse must be keenly aware of aseptic practices in order to maintain the sterile field at all times. The best source of information is contained in the current *AORN Standards, Recommended Practices, and Guidelines,* published annually to provide the best evidence-based practices. These principles are the basis for accepted OR protocol and a basis for all hospital policies and procedures.

Implants

A number of implants are used in surgery today. There are many orthopedic implants such as hip and knee components, screws, plates, rods, cages, and accessory items. There also are bone and tissue implants; these include bone grafts, bone pieces, tendons, skin, and other tissues. Other specialties use implants as well. These items are all governed by the FDA, which has strict guidelines for properly documenting and tracking implanted devices. They require that records be kept regarding the date of receipt of implants. Storage requirements, including temperature logs, also must be documented. The information required regarding implantation is significant. Documentation should include the patient's permanent record, the perioperative nurse's notes, and the implant log. Hospitals must be able to track each implanted tissue or device, should there be a recall of the product. The information should include the lot number, manufacturer, serial number, size and type, and anatomic position of the implant (Rothrock, 2003).

The nurse must ensure that all implants are sterile, preferably sterilized ahead of time. According to the AORN Recommended Practices for Sterilization in the Perioperative Practice Setting (AORN, 2006), flash sterilization should not be used for implantable devices. If an implantable device must be sterilized at a health care facility, a biological indicator should be run with the sterilizer load, and the implant should remain quarantined until the results of the biological indicator are obtained. If an implant must be flashed in an emergency situation, a rapid-action biological monitoring device should be used, along with a class V chemical integrator. The implant should not be released for use until the rapid-action biological indicator provides a negative result. After the negative result is obtained, the implant may be released for immediate use. If the implant is not used, it cannot be resterilized for future use.

Documentation of All Nursing Interventions

Documentation in the patient's medical record is critical to patient care. The documentation is how caregivers communicate with one another. It also is the legal record of the patient's care. Generally, it is accepted that "if it isn't documented, it wasn't done." All patient interactions should be documented in the record.

The circulating nurse must document activities performed to achieve the expected outcome. In perioperative nursing, the *Perioperative Nursing Data Set* (PNDS) is the recognized standard language, and its use is encouraged. The circulating nurse should document:

- preoperative history and physical;
- lab reports;
- consents;
- patient identification and site verification;
- significant intraoperative times;
- patient condition on receipt and transfer;
- method of transport;
- level of consciousness;
- patient position during surgery;
- skin condition;
- site preparation;
- intravenous site and specifics regarding fluids and type of needle;
- medications;

- type of anesthesia;
- tourniquet specifics;
- estimated blood loss;
- sponge, instrument, and sharps count results;
- surgical procedure performed;
- equipment used, such as lasers and electrosurgical units;
- implants;
- specimens and cultures;
- use of x-rays;
- site and type of drains;
- wound classifications;
- dressing applied;
- any unusual events; and
- all personnel in the room and their times of entry and exit.

Environmental Factors

The main focus of environmental control (e.g., temperature, humidity, air exchanges) is infection control, occupant comfort, and patient normothermia, the greatest of these being infection control. The greatest amount of bacteria found in the OR comes from the surgical team and is a result of their activities before and during surgery (U.S. Department of Veteran Affairs, 2005). Because the surgical team at the sterile field often has on layers of heavy clothing and they stand under lights and where medical machines put out heat, they often complain of being warm. Thus, the OR is kept cooler. The humidity must be kept low to keep the sterile supplies from sweating. The number of air exchanges has been established to prevent infection by moving air into and out of the OR rather quickly.

There are specific recommendations for environmental control in the OR. The American Institute of Architects (AIA) has design guidelines that direct those environmental factors. They recommend 15 air changes per hour of supply air for an OR, and 20% of that supply must be outdoor air (Murphy, 2006).

Several agencies specify recommended settings for environmental control of ORs. The American Society of Heating, Refrigeration, and Air Conditioning Engineers (ASHRAE) has standards for ORs for temperature, humidity, and air exchanges (Murphy, 2006). They state that room temperature should range from 68° to 75° F (20° to 24° C) with humidity of 30% to 60% (Murphy, 2006). The AIA recommends a temperature of 68° to 73° F (20° to 23° C) with a humidity of 30% to 60% (Murphy, 2006).

Hospital staff generally view noise as a day-to-day annoyance that must be tolerated. However, to patients and even some clinical staff, that noise can be very negative. This is not a new problem. Florence Nightingale identified noise as a very serious insult to patients as well as a deterrent to healing (Mazer, 2005). In 1972, the U.S. Congress passed the Noise Control Act and the Environmental Protection Agency (EPA) formed the EPA Office of Noise Abatement and Control (Mazer, 2005). OSHA calls noise simply "unwanted sound" and has stated that excessive noise can hinder communication, limit performance, and have other health impacts (Mazer, 2005). In a research study on noise, John Hopkins University researchers reported that excessive noise leads to stressed workers, raises the risk of errors, and can interfere with healing and recovery (ASHA, 2006).

The noise level of the OR should be considered. Certainly, the noise level is often high. There is the noise of staff asking for supplies and instruments. Today, many newer ORs have piped in music and older ones have small stereo systems or DVD players. Patients are bombarded by sounds that are loud and sometimes unfamiliar, and thus more disturbing to them. There is the constant ringing of the telephone, pagers and cell phones, medical alarms, fire alarms, and intercom announcements and paging. Imagine the sound of a scrub person tossing a weighted vaginal speculum into the basin while waiting for water. These are sounds that have been heard in ORs. And people tend to just talk louder as it gets noisier, such as at a crowded social gathering.

In today's climate of patient safety, the nurse must recognize that excessive noise can definitely contribute to errors. He or she can lead others to reduce the noise level in the surgical suite by considering steps that can be taken to reduce the noise. Hospitals can reduce the noise with a concerted effort. Many hospitals have practically eliminated overhead paging. Others have provided nurses with portable telephones that can be placed on vibrate. Some have small handheld devices that eliminate the need for paging and ringing phones. Sometimes just raising the awareness of staff members can help reduce the noise level.

In the OR, the perioperative nurse must be aware of noise and work to control that noise. The music should be appropriate to the listener. Certainly, it should be discontinued at the request of the patient or any health care team member. The OR should be as quiet as possible, particularly during anesthesia induction and emergence. Only necessary talking should take place, and then at low levels. Counting should be done quietly. Little things need to be considered: the crushing of surgical wrapping paper; the clatter of instruments; objects being rolled across the floor; the noise of the suction running; and continuous monitor beeps (Phillips, 2004). The perioperative nurse should lead the surgical team to reduce as much noise as possible.

Selecting, Cleaning, Packaging, Sterilizing, and Disinfecting Methods

Cleaning, disinfection, and sterilization are the processes by which items are rendered sterile and thus usable for surgery. Instruments can be cleaned manually or by washer-sterilizer or washer-decontaminator. The purpose of cleaning is to remove bioburden (residual blood and debris) before sterilization or disinfection. Ultrasonic cleaners are also available. The perioperative nurse must consider what is to be cleaned. Delicate eye instruments might be best cleaned by hand, while instruments with a heavy bioburden, such as total hip instruments, can be cleaned best through an automated process.

There are three classifications of patient care items: critical items that must be sterile because they enter a sterile area on a patient; semi-critical items that come into contact with non-intact skin and mucous membranes that require high-level disinfection; and non-critical items that contact only intact skin.

There are three levels of disinfection. High-level disinfection kills all bacteria, viruses, and fungi. It may kill spores if contact is long enough. Intermediate disinfection kills most bacteria, viruses, and fungi. Low-level disinfection kills most vegetative bacteria, fungi, and least resistant viruses. The nurse must know what instrument or equipment is to be disinfected because items require different levels of disinfection (Phillip, 2004). The nurse must select the appropriate method each time. There are chemical disinfectants and physical disinfectants. Again, the nurse must understand the properties of the item to be disinfected and the level of disinfection required before selecting an appropriate method. These are the criteria that will lead to proper selection.

As stated, critical items must be sterile and therefore require sterilization. There are several methods of sterilization: thermal, steam under pressure (i.e., moist heat) or hot air (i.e., dry heat); chemical, ethylene oxide, formaldehyde, hydrogen peroxide, ozone gas, acetic acid, gluteraldehyde solutions, and peracetic acid; and radiation, microwave, or x-ray. Sterilization indicates that the product has been exposed to the parameters of sterilization, which are considered to signify the reliability of the process. These parameters include:

- temperature;
- humidity/moisture/hydration;
- time;
- purity of the sterilizing agent;
- saturation/penetration; and
- capability of the sterilizer and position of items within the chamber (Phillips, 2004).

Performing and Documenting Sterilization Procedures

All personnel performing sterilization must have a grasp of the principles of sterilization. They must understand how all equipment works and know the methods used to monitor the process. Work practices of sterilization are strictly enforced by an institution's policies and procedures that are based on accepted principles and evidence-based practice. Policies and procedures should cover:

- decontamination of all reusable items;
- packaging and labeling systems;
- loading and unloading the sterilizer;
- operating the sterilizer;
- monitoring and maintaining record of sterilization;
- adhering to safety precautions;
- storing sterile items;
- handling sterile items; and
- tracking and recalling items (Phillips, 2004).

While it is accepted that items are flashed only during an emergency, records must be maintained to document that the parameters of sterilization were met whenever an instrument is "flashed."

Conducting and Documenting Biological Monitoring

Assurance that sterilization has occurred can only be provided though a biological indicator. A biological indicator is a preparation of living spores that are resistant to the sterilizing agent. The biological unit is exposed to the sterilant. Then that biological and an unprocessed biological unit from the same lot number are incubated for the same period of time. If the processed indicator shows no growth and the processed indicator shows growth, sterilization has occurred. Some hospitals use biologicals every day, and others use them in every load. This depends on the hospital's policy regarding biologicals. Every load of implantables should be monitored, and the implant should not be used until a negative reading occurs. All test results are maintained as a permanent record so items can be recalled if needed (Philips, 2004).

Conducting and Documenting Chemical Monitoring

Chemical indicators are used on the inside and outside of sterile packages. External indicators include paper, tape, labels, or paper strips. They are clearly visible on the outside of every package. The internal indicator is placed inside of the package. The nurse must examine the indicator to determine if the package contents have been exposed to the parameters of sterilization. These indicators do not ensure sterility. They only show that the package has been exposed to the sterilization parameters. If the parameters of sterilization have not been met, the item must not be considered sterile.

Monitoring and Documenting Package Integrity

Each package of sterile items must be maintained in acceptable condition—dry and at the appropriate temperature. When a package is placed on a shelf to indicate it is sterile and ready for use, the package should be inspected. When the item is presented to the sterile field, the packaging is inspected. The nurse must ensure the package integrity to assume that the item is sterile. The nurse inspects the package for damage—holes, tears, or any aberration to the package. If the package integrity is breached, the package is considered unsterile and a new package must be obtained.

Please refer to Chapter 6: Cleaning, Disinfecting, Packaging, and Sterilizing for a complete discussion on these topics.

Summary

This chapter has dealt with the task statement: Management of Personnel, Services, and Materials. The perioperative nurse has a great deal of responsibility for patient safety. Effective management of these issues will be a very good beginning to providing the patient a safe and effective visit to the OR for a surgical procedure. The nurse must always remember that he or she is the patient's advocate during the surgical journey. The nurse speaks for the patient when he or she is unable to do so. The work of the perioperative nurse begins before the patient arrives in the OR as the nurse prepares for personnel, services, and materials.

The nurse follows established policies and procedures of the institution as well as standards, recommended practices, and guidelines from AORN. These are the framework for professional perioperative practice established by perioperative leaders across the country. The management of personnel, supplies, and materials requires critical thinking skills as well as knowing policies and guidelines. The management by the perioperative nurse is continued through surgery and into the postoperative phase to ensure a safe and effective surgical experience. As with all that the nurse does, the goal of managing these aspects of care is a safe and effective patient outcome.

Case Study

It is 11:30 PM on a Friday night. Mr. K is a 57-year-old male in the emergency department (ED). (This hospital has 5 operating rooms). He has been in a motorcycle accident and has been in the ED for several hours. He has had a computed tomography (CT) scan and x-rays. The CT showed bleeding from the spleen. The ED physician is going to observe Mr. K. However, when the radiology technician stands Mr. K up for a chest x-ray, he passes out. He is cold and clammy and very pale. His blood pressure is 70/40. He is rushed back to the ED. His blood pressure is maintained by rapid infusion of packed red blood cells. When the ED physician discovers Mr. K takes warfarin (Coumadin) regularly for his atrial fibrillation, he calls in the trauma surgeon. The trauma surgeon calls in the OR team for surgery as soon as possible.

When BL, the perioperative nurse on call, arrives at the hospital for surgery, he goes by the ED to check on Mr. K and to get an idea of what to expect. BL gets a report and goes to the OR to begin preparing for the case.

Discussion Points for Case Study

1. BL, the perioperative nurse, is the only RN on call. There will be one surgical technologist who will scrub. Because two nurses were working with the blood infusion in the ED, BL anticipates that he might have difficulty handling the needs of the anesthesiologist and the scrub technician at once. What could the nurse do to proactively be ready for this difficulty?

2. When Mr. K is moved to the OR bed, he immediately converts his sinus rhythm to ventricular tachycardia. What is a possible reason for this conversion? What treatment is required? What dysrhythmia follows if the ventricular tachycardia is not converted to sinus rhythm?

3. What other blood products might BL expect to need for this case?

4. What are additional supplies that the nurse might bring to the operating room to be prepared for this case?

5. What piece of equipment should the nurse set up ahead of time?

6. Are there outside services that should be requested to be present?

7. Mr. K had a large meal at 7:00 PM. It is now 11:30 PM. What precautions should the perioperative nurse take?

8. Is there an emergency piece of equipment that the nurse should provide based on Mr. K's cardiac history?

9. Discuss the importance of normothermia and consequences of inadvertent hypothermia? Describe methods that the surgical team can use to prevent hypothermia.

10. Mr. K has survived the surgery and is in the intensive care unit. On Sunday BL, the nurse, runs into a motorcycling buddy of Mr. K's at the big weekend motorcycle event. Mr. K's buddy seeks out BL to see how Mr. K is doing and what actually happened. What is the appropriate way for BL to handle this?

Responses to consider:

1. Because he is hemorrhaging severely from his spleen, adequate fluid resuscitation and blood product administration is essential to a positive outcome for Mr. K. The nurse, BL, must arrange to have the needed assistance and use his critical thinking skills to arrange for assistance that he might need. He has several options. Assuming that there is no back-up perioperative OR nurse on call, the best option is to call the postanesthesia care unit (PACU) RN on call to come in now to assist him. He might also call the nursing supervisor and ask him or her for assistance. Perhaps the ED is not too busy and can send an RN to assist with fluid resuscitation and administration of blood products. He might also call the administrative person on call for the operating room.

   BL also has an opportunity to create improvement for this operating room for future cases. He should discuss this situation with the surgical services administrator or operating room manager. He can offer to lead a team to identify potential solutions and make a recommendation to administration so that a plan can be developed to handle any future situations such as this. Then should an event of this nature occur again, the perioperative nurse will have a plan to follow to arrange for appropriate assistance.

2. Mr. K most likely has hypovolemia from the hemorrhaging and excessive blood loss. He may be in hypovolemic shock and the ventricular tachycardia can lead to death. The nurse must provide the defibrillator so Mr. K can be given a shock to convert his rhythm. Without a "shock," the ventricular tachycardia will progress to ventricular fibrillation, which if untreated is fatal.

3. In addition to fluid replacement volume with intravenous fluids, the nurse can expect Mr. K to receive additional whole blood, plasma expanders, and packed cells.

4. Due to severe hemorrhaging from the spleen, the nurse should have extra supplies of intravenous fluids and volume expanders, blood pump, fluid and warmer, blood filters, laparotomy pads, and raytec sponges.

5. Because the hospital is a small hospital and is not a trauma center, they do not have a perfusionist on staff. They have a contracted service that provides their autologous blood salvage. The "cell saver" (i.e., autologous blood salvage machine) should be set up. The surgical team can begin collecting blood from Mr. K's abdominal cavity for autotransfusion prior to the arrival of the "cell saver" personnel. Then there will be fluid to prepare and return to Mr. K.

6. The nurse should notify the "cell saver" personnel that there is a trauma coming to surgery and their services will be needed as soon as possible for autologous blood salvage and transfusion.

7. Suction should be set up and readily available due to Mr. K's full stomach and the possibility for vomiting and aspiration. The nurse also should consider having a nasogastric tube available for insertion.

8. Due to Mr. K's chronic atrial fibrillation, the nurse should arrange to have the defibrillator available. There may be need for cardioversion at some point during or after the case. Also Mr. K is prone to cardiac dysrhythmia due to severe fluid loss.

9. It is important for the surgical team to attempt to maintain normothermia. The patient might be expected to develop hypothermia during surgery. He will have a large incision during his surgery for an exploratory laparotomy. There will be irrigation fluids and the OR will provide a cooler than normal ambient temperature for Mr. K. Inadvertent intraoperative hypothermia can lead to a number of different complications. These include dysrhythmia, increased potential for infection, coagulopathy, and delayed drug excretion.

   There are a number of steps that can be taken to help maintain normothermia. These include: elevating the room temperature; limiting skin exposure during positioning and skin preparation; using a patient warming system that circulates warm water through pads on which the patient lies; using fluid warming devices for irrigation fluids as well as intravenous fluids and blood, and using forced air warming blankets that are placed on the patient.

10. The nurse must adhere to the Health Insurance Portability and Accountability Act (HIPAA) regulations. The HIPAA regulations require that the nurse protect the personal health information of Mr. K. The nurse must explain that he is unable to discuss Mr. K's health with him and suggest that "the buddy" call Mr. K's family.

Suggested Learning Activities

- Seek additional information regarding communication skills.
- Review the current JCAHO National Patient Safety Goals.
- Review AORN's Patient Safety web site.
- Review the current AORN recommended practices related to patient safety.
- Review AORN's Workplace Safety link at www.aorn.org.
- Review principles of positioning.
- Discuss basic management skills.
- Review the many documents on the JCAHO web site (www.jointcommission.org).
- Review the ANA Code of Ethics for Nurses with Explications for Perioperative Nursing in the current edition of AORN's *Standards, Recommended Practices, and Guidelines.*
- Review your state's nurse practice act.
- Review Health Insurance Portability and Accountability Act regulations.
- Discuss quality improvement activities within your facility.
- Review patients' rights and responsibilities at your institution.
- Review aseptic technique.
- Discuss biological and chemical monitoring with the central sterilization department.

Chapter 9
Professional Accountability

Cecil A. King, RN, MS, CNOR

According to the American Nurses Association (ANA), "The nursing profession contracts with society to promote health, to do no harm, and to respond with skill and caring when change, birth, illness, disease, or death is experienced" (ANA, 2004). This statement alludes to nursing as being accountable to society as a profession and by virtue of licensure, as having a social responsibility for which the profession individually and collectively is held responsible. A profession acquires meaning in terms of its relationship with society. The professional skills and services that are needed by a profession are driven by the needs of the society it serves. The profession of nursing is based on this social contract that distinguishes professional rights and responsibilities and establishes societal accountability. Professional nursing, through self-regulation, is accountable for ensuring its individual nurses act in the public's best interest during the course of providing nursing services. (ANA, 2003).

Professional accountability is inherent to any profession. Those entering the profession of nursing are held accountable to the profession, to the public, and to oneself for the practice of nursing appropriate to one's education, experience, and situation. Accountability is a multi-faceted concept and implies that one also has a responsibility or an obligation to do or not do something. The perioperative nurse's primary commitment is the patient; because of this nurse-patient relationship, there is an obligation on the part of the nurse to provide safe, professional, and ethical care in a non-judgmental manner.

Accountability is the quality of being responsible. State nurse practice acts and nursing practice standards provide the foundation for the registered nurse's (RN) professional accountability. Professional practice standards reflect the values and priorities of the profession. Standards are authoritative affirmations that describe the responsibilities for which the perioperative nurse is accountable and provide direction and a means by which to evaluate professional nursing practice (AORN, 2006). Standards of practice describe what is considered to be a minimal level of competency as demonstrated by the critical thinking model we know as the nursing process (i.e., assessment, diagnosis, outcome identification, planning, implementation, and evaluation).

The ANA has developed generic standards that apply across specialties and has identified emerging themes that are fundamental to many standards of practice that span across practice settings:

- age-appropriate, culturally and ethnically sensitive care;
- maintaining a safe environment of care;
- patient education;
- providing continuity of care;
- coordinating care across setting and providers;
- information management;
- effective communication; and
- technology utilization (ANA, 2004).

Practice standards, regulations, and statutes govern the practice of professional nursing. These various sets of guidelines have been developed to protect and promote the welfare of the patients nurses serve. "Registered nurses are accountable for their professional actions to themselves, their patients, their peers, and, ultimately, to society" (ANA, 2005). The professional nurse's responsibilities are expressed by the ANA's *Nursing Scope and Standards of Practice* (ANA, 2004), the *Code of Ethics for Nurses with Interpretive Statements* (ANA, 2001), the Association of periOperative Registered Nurses' (AORN) *Standards, Recommended Practices, and Guidelines* (AORN, 2006), and AORN's Explications for Perioperative Nursing (AORN, 2006). Together these documents provide a framework of the perioperative nurse's accountability and responsibility to the public, other health care providers, and the profession of nursing. This chapter allows perioperative nurses to assess their professional conduct and use recommendations to develop and maintain professional accountability.

Learning Objectives

Professional registered nurses preparing for the certification exam in perioperative nursing should include the areas of requisite knowledge and skills to establish and maintain professional accountability. Upon completion of this chapter, the individual should be able to:

1. Discuss nursing professional accountability to the patient, profession, and public.

Task/Knowledge/Skill Statements

Assess personal limitations and seek assistance as needed

- Transcultural nursing theory (e.g., cultural and ethnic influences; family patterns; spiritually and related practices)
- Community and instructional resources
- Surgical procedure
- Pharmacology and anesthetic agents
- Principles of patient safety
- Principles of positioning
- Ergonomics and body mechanics (e.g., patient/equipment)
- Basic management techniques and delegation
- Regulatory standards and voluntary guidelines (e.g., AORN *Standards, Recommended Practices and Guidelines*; OSHA; JCAHO; ANA Code of Ethics for Nurses with Explications for Perioperative Nurses; state Nurse Practice Act)
- Responsibilities regarding impaired and/or disruptive behavior (e.g., patient/family; multidisciplinary health care team members)
- Clinical privileges
- Resources for professional growth (e.g., *Perioperative Nursing Data Set* [PNDS]; computer skills)

Identify and report impaired/disruptive behavior of inpatients, their family, and/or multidisciplinary health care team

- Health assessment techniques
- Transcultural nursing theory (e.g., cultural and ethnic influences; family patterns; spiritually and related practices)
- Behavioral responses to the surgical experience
- Patient rights and responsibilities
- Legal responsibilities and implications for patient care
- Interviewing techniques (e.g., patient/family)
- Reporting techniques to multidisciplinary health care providers (e.g., critical lab values, medical condition, medications; allergies; implants/implantable devices; hand off; read back verbal orders; communication barriers)
- Basic management techniques and delegation
- Regulatory standards and voluntary guidelines (e.g., AORN *Standards, Recommended Practices and Guidelines*; OSHA; JCAHO; ANA Code of Ethics for Nurses with Explications for Perioperative Nurses; state Nurse Practice Act)
- Responsibilities regarding impaired and/or disruptive behavior (e.g., patient/family; multidisciplinary health care team members)

Uphold and act upon ethical and professional standards

- Patient rights and responsibilities
- Legal responsibilities and implications for patient care
- Principles of patient safety
- Principles of patients' rights
- Regulatory standards and voluntary guidelines (e.g., AORN *Standards, Recommended Practices and Guidelines*; OSHA; JCAHO; AND Coded of Ethics for Nurses with Explications for Perioperative →

2. Differentiate between accountability and responsibility.

3. Describe three aspects of professional accountability.

4. Identify the nursing process as the demonstrated foundation of critical thinking in the practice of professional nursing.

5. Identify the individual nurse's reasonability for professional growth and performance improvement.

6. Describe the core competency of professional perioperative nursing within the domains of the *Perioperative Nursing Data Set* (PNDS).

Accountability and Responsibility

Nursing professional accountability and ethical obligations are made explicit in the nine provisions of the *Code of Ethics for Nurses* (ANA, 2001). The first three provisions describe the primary responsibility of nursing is to provide care to patients and their family; the second three address the boundaries of duty and loyalty; and the later three describe the nursing profession's duties to society. Provision four in the *Code of Ethics* reads: "The nurse is responsible and accountable for individual nursing practice and determines the appropriate delegation of tasks consistent with the nurse's obligation to provide optimum patient care" (ANA , 2001). Perioperative nurses are accountable for judgments made and actions taken in the course of their practice. Nurses are accountable to the profession and the public to maintain licensure and continually acquire knowledge and skills about new treatments and technology.

Assess Personal Limitations and Seek Assistance As Needed

Perioperative nurses are continually challenged by the

Task/Knowledge/Skill Statements

Nurses; state Nurse Practice Act)
- Responsibilities regarding impaired and/or disruptive behavior (e.g., patient/family; multidisciplinary health care team members)
- Clinical privileges
- Resources for professional growth (e.g., *Perioperative Nursing Data Set* [PNDS]; computer skills)
- Nursing research and evidence-based practice

Identify and utilize resources for professional growth

- Patient rights and responsibilities
- Legal responsibilities and implications for patient care
- Principles of patient safety
- Principles of patients' rights
- Communication theories and techniques (e.g., patient/family)
- Basic management techniques and delegation
- Regulatory standards and voluntary guidelines (e.g., AORN *Standards, Recommended Practices and Guidelines*; OSHA; JCAHO; ANA Code of Ethics for Nurses with Explications for Perioperative Nurses; state Nurse Practice Act)
- Responsibilities regarding impaired and/or disruptive behavior (e.g., patient/family; multidisciplinary health care team members)
- Clinical privileges
- Resources for professional growth (e.g., *Perioperative Nursing Data Set* [PNDS]; computer skills)
- Nursing research and evidence-based practice

Participate in quality improvement activities

- Community and instructional resources
- Expected outcomes related to identified interventions
- Ergonomics and body mechanics (e.g., patient/equipment)
- Requirements of handling specimens
- Documentation of all nursing interventions
- Standard and transmission-based precautions
- Documentation of sterilization, biological and chemical monitoring
- Selecting cleaning, packaging, sterilizing and disinfecting methods
- Performing and documenting disinfection procedures for equipment and instruments
- Performing and documenting sterilization procedures
- Conducting and documenting biological monitoring
- Principles of product evaluation and cost containment
- Quality improvement principles
- Acquisition processes for equipment, supplies, and personnel
- Basic management techniques and delegation
- Regulatory standards and voluntary guidelines (e.g., AORN *Standards, Recommended Practices and Guidelines*; OSHA; JCAHO; ANA Code of Ethics for Nurses with Explications for Perioperative Nurses; state Nurse Practice Act)
- Resources for professional growth (e.g., *Perioperative Nursing Data Set* [PNDS]; computer skills)
- Nursing research and evidence-based practice

ever progressive and changing technology and milieu of surgery and perioperative services. Therefore, nurses are responsible for taking measures to continue their specific knowledge acquisition and assessing individual competence as part of their commitment to lifelong learning. Nurses develop and maintain current knowledge and skills by actively seeking opportunities for professional growth and performance improvement activities (e.g., certification). The science of nursing is based on critical thinking as demonstrated by application of the nursing process. The following core standards of practice and sub-activities of implementation make up the steps in the critical thinking process known as the nursing process and are foundational to professional nursing practice:

1. Assessment
2. Diagnosis
3. Outcomes identification
4. Planning
5. Implementation:
   a. Coordination of care
   b. Health teaching and health promotion
   c. Consultation
   d. Prescriptive authority and treatment
6. Evaluation (ANA, 2004)

Perioperative nurses are not only responsible for knowing their own level of knowledge and skills, but are also equally responsible for the outcomes of tasks they delegate. Therefore, it is imperative for the professional nurse to know the competency level of those to whom tasks are delegated. Just as there are five "rights" of medication administration, there are five "rights" of delegation, including:

- right task,
- right circumstance,
- right person,
- right communication, and

- right level of supervision (VanCura & Gunchick, 1997).

Nursing activities such as assessment, patient outcome identification, planning, and evaluation cannot be delegated. The following factors should be taken into consideration when delegating certain nursing activities to assistive personnel:

- overall patient condition, complexity, and/or acuity;
- complexity of the skills required to perform the delegated activity or procedure;
- predictability of achieving the desired outcome;
- knowledge that the person you are delegating to has demonstrated competency (competency within this context means that the person has the knowledge, skills, and professional attitude to safely carry out the delegation);
- staffing ratios, RN to assistive personnel; and
- amount of supervision required and the RN's ability to provide it (AORN, 2006).

The fifth provision the *Code of Ethics for Nurses with Interpretive Statements* states that "The nurse owes the same duties to self as to others, including the responsibility to preserve integrity and safety, to maintain competence, and to continue personal and professional growth" (ANA, 2001). This statement recognizes the individual nurse's professional (and ethical) obligation to self in sustaining lifelong learning, competency (e.g., clinical, technical, information literacy), one's personal and professional values, and integrity. Having a duty to oneself reveals the personhood of the nurse and accentuates the nurse's primary duty to oneself as being honest with oneself and frank about individual strengthens and weaknesses.

The nurse demonstrates duty to self by continuing personal and professional growth that includes seeking opportunities for knowledge and skill acquisition to address weaknesses identified as part of one's annual and ongoing performance review. The practice of perioperative nursing requires the practitioner to have a broad knowledge base and skills, as well as the ability to collaborate effectively with other health care providers. As a professional, the perioperative RN has an obligation to establish and maintain the appropriate level of knowledge, skills, and competency required to be able to care safely for the surgical patient.

The art and science of professional nursing practice involves both the behavioral and physical sciences, which are in a constant state of change and progress. To function safely in the dynamic perioperative environment and to be able to achieve desirable patient outcomes, the nurse has a professional responsibility to participate in continuing education and professional development. The professional nurse is accountable to oneself, the profession, and society for maintaining his or her individual competency. Some of the methods by which the individual professional nurse may maintain current and practical knowledge and competence include the following.

- Orientation—including the identification of individual learning needs based on the competencies required by a particular practice setting (e.g., hospital, ambulatory center, free-standing centers), the population served, and/or the procedures performed (e.g., bariatrics, pediatrics, trauma).

- Competency validation—competency is comprised of three elements: 1) knowledge, 2) psychomotor skills, and 3) professional attitude or one's ability to perform according to facility policy, procedure, and standards of practice (e.g., Joint Commission on Accreditation of Healthcare Organizations [JCAHO], AORN). Competency may be developed by a facility of employment related to a specific procedure or technology, such as laser surgery, or may refer to those developed by our professional associations (e.g., Competency Statements in Perioperative Nursing [AORN, 2006]).

- Professional goals and objectives—setting goals and developing a professional development plan as part of your annual performance and peer review (e.g., certification, leadership roles, clinical ladders, advanced degrees).

- Continuing education—both formal and informal methods of increasing one's knowledge (e.g., reading professional journals, attending in-service programs and professional conferences, participating in home study or self-study educational modules).

The ultimate goal of perioperative professional nursing is to achieve desired patient outcomes. Patient outcomes are those measurable physiologic and psychosocial patient responses to nursing interventions attributed to collegial collaboration and independent nursing activities. It is this element of independent nursing practice that makes it possible for nurses to have a scope of practice recognized by state governments and legitimized by licensure. AORN's *Perioperative Nursing Data Set* (Beyea, 2002) is an empirically validated data set of patient outcomes with corresponding nursing interventions and activities that explicate those nursing activities that differentiates perioperative nurses from other professionals. One of the PNDS outcome statements specifically states that ". . . the patient is the recipient of competent and ethical care within legal standards of care" (Beyea, 2002). The outcome statement implies that the RN is responsible for maintaining competency through continual education and competency validation.

It is the individual responsibility of the nurse to identify deficits and limitations in knowledge and skill and develop a correction plan of action. Should such an instance occur in an immediate patient care situation (e.g., the nurse does not know how to use a piece of equipment), it is the nurse's personal and professional responsibility to seek collaboration and consultation in the operation of the equipment, including the manufacturer's documented instructions. The same is true as it relates to facility of employment policy and procedure. It is the individual's responsibility to know facility policy and procedure and seek clarification and instruction when one does not understand the expectation of the one's employer.

AORN has delineated specific perioperative core competencies within the domains of the Perioperative Patient Care Model. Those AORN perioperative competency statements are as follows:

- **Safety**—"The perioperative registered nurse demonstrates the ability to establish an environment of safety for the surgical patient."

- **Physiologic**—"The perioperative registered nurse demonstrates the ability to assess, diagnose, implement, and evaluate treatments and procedures that contribute to the physiological stability of the surgical patient."

- **Behavioral Responses: Knowledge**—"The perioperative registered nurse demonstrates knowledge about the psychologic, sociologic, and spiritual responses of patients and their families to the operative or other invasive procedure, including participation of patient in their recovery."

- **Behavioral Responses: Patient and Family Rights/Ethics**—"The perioperative registered nurse supports patients' rights and ethics by delivering consistent, competent, and ethical care, within legal standards of practice, while maintaining privacy and support of the patient's value system."

- **Health System Outcomes**—"The perioperative registered nurse demonstrates knowledge of the health system environment and administrative issues that impact job performance, patient safety, and ethical considerations." (AORN, 2006).

Competent performance is commonly assessed as a dimension on one's annual performance evaluation. Elements of what constitutes competent performance include:

- being observed by a peer or one's supervisor demonstrating a specific skill set (e.g., competent to position as evidenced by the patient being free from injury related to positioning);
- compliance with local, state, and federal regulations;
- appropriate delegation to competent and appropriate assistive personnel;
- practicing accordingly within one's legal scope of practice and ethical codes;
- confirming clinician privileges;
- certification (e.g., CNOR, CRNFA) as a mechanism that may demonstrate competency; and
- performing the role of patient advocate and intervening to protect the patient from physical or psychological harm (Beyea, 2002).

Identify and Report Impaired/Disruptive Behavior of Inpatients, Their Family, and/or Multidisciplinary Health Care Team

The third provision of the *Code of Ethics for Nurses* gives direction to the perioperative nurse in matters of patient advocacy: "The nurse promotes, advocates for and strives to protect the health, safety, and rights of the patient" (ANA, 2001). Patient advocacy in its broadest sense implies that the nurse supports patient's rights and acts on behalf of the patient. The function of patient advocacy is especially pertinent to the care of the patient in surgery when the patient is most vulnerable and unable to act on his or her own behalf. The perioperative nurse has both a legal and an ethical obligation to protect patients from incompetent, unethical, or illegal practices by complying with facility policies, state and federal regulations (e.g., department of health, Occupational Safety and Health Administration [OSHA], state nurse practice acts), and national standards as set forth by accrediting agencies and professional associations (e.g., JCAHO, AORN, Centers for Disease Control and Prevention [CDC]).

Nurse should know how to verify clinicians' privileges and credentials (Beyea, 2002). In addition to one's individual accountability for compliance and competency, the nurse has a professional responsibility to enact appropriate reporting mechanisms regarding instances of incompetent, unethical, illegal, or impaired practice by any member of the health care team or any action or inaction on the part of others (i.e., either individuals or health care systems or organizational processes) that jeopardize the best interest of the patient or pose potential harm to the patient and/or employee of the organization. Organizations should have mechanisms in place that support reporting of incompetent, unethical, illegal, or impaired practice without fear of retribution or reprisal (e.g., anonymous reporting) (ANA, 2001).

Nurses have a four-fold responsibility to protect the patient, the public, the impaired provider, and the profession from harm any time a colleague may be impaired.

We customarily think of an impaired provider as one with the illness of substance abuse or addiction, but it may be due to any mental or physical illness or personal circumstance that interferes with one's ability to safely perform the duties of his or her job. As when any illness impedes one's ability to function, the same caring, compassion, and appropriate intervention should be extended to those impaired. When a nurse suspects that a member of the health care team or any colleague may be impaired, the nurse has an ethical and professional responsibility to take action that both protects patients and provides appropriate intervention to the impaired colleague.

Any time the nurse is addressing questionable practice (e.g., incompetent, unethical, illegal, impaired practice), such action usually begins in consultation with one's immediate supervisor. The nurse should follow facility policies as well as guidelines delineated by the profession (e.g., state board of nursing) to assist colleagues whose practice is compromised by mental or physical illness or personal circumstances. This includes assistance with treatment, counseling and access to just institutional and legal processes, and the return to work of those who have sought appropriate assistance and are ready to resume their professional duties (ANA, 2001).

Uphold and Act Upon Ethical and Professional Standards

Professional standards, regulations, and statutes govern the practice of professional nursing. These various guidelines exist to provide direction to the profession and to protect and promote optimal patient care. The RN is expected to integrate these professional standards and the provisions of the *Code of Ethics for Nurses* (ANA, 2001) in all areas of practice. The ANA Code and AORN's Explications for Perioperative Nursing (AORN, 2006) make explicit the values and ethical obligations of the professional nurse. "It is the profession's nonnegotiable ethical standard" (ANA, 2001). Professional codes of ethics are the primary identifying mark of a profession that spell out the norms of behavior and the ethical norms or morality of a profession.

Ethical nursing care is care delivered in a manner that preserves the dignity of, respect for, and rights of the individual patient. Nursing has an ethical obligation in the role of patient advocate to operate as the patient's moral agent. There are primarily three ethical principles that underpin the morality of nursing:

- autonomy, which is the respect for personhood and the patient's right to self-determination (e.g., informed consent);
- beneficence, which is doing good; and
- nonmaleficence, which is to do no harm—as it is not adequate to merely do good, but necessary to weigh proportionally the probability of benefit to doing no harm (AORN, 2004).

The ethical metaparadigm for the nursing profession is social reasonability, autonomy or respect for personhood, nonmaleficence, and justice as fairness (Silva & Ludwick, 2006).

The ability to conduct ethical examinations is a significant component of professional nursing practice. When facing a clinical issue lacking sound scientific evidence to guide one's conduct, one may be facing an ethical issue in determining what one ought to do. Perioperative nurses should be able to recognize an ethical dilemma and use the ANA *Code of Ethics for Nurses* (ANA, 2001) and AORN's Explications for Perioperative Nursing (AORN, 2006) as guidelines in determining how to resolve the dilemma. A critical aspect, as well as the key underpinning the nurse's ethical responsibility to the patient, is the protection of patients' rights, in addition to the right to safe and competent care. As the patient's moral agent, the professional nurse employs practice standards to protect the health, safety, and rights of the patient. This need for patient moral agency emerges from the impact of illness compounded with the perioperative contextual features that affect the patient's ability to act on his or her own behalf.

The following principles outline the role of the nurse in providing ethical patient care during the perioperative period.

- The RN is responsible for safeguarding the patient's confidentiality and dignity. In the perioperative setting, this may include limiting access to the OR schedule; confining conversations about the patient's care to the OR suite and conversing only with those involved in the care of the patient; minimizing exposure of the patient's body during positioning and prepping, and following the Recommended Practices for Traffic Patterns in the Perioperative Practice Setting (AORN, 2006).

- Professional nurses have an ethical obligation to provide care without regard to race, gender, sexual orientation, creed, or cultural beliefs.

- Care must be provided to the patient and family (however the patient defines his or her family) by including them in decisions affecting the patient's health care, in providing care and teaching, and at the same time respecting the patient's autonomy, dignity, and right to self-determination.

- Nurses may find themselves in difficult or uncomfortable situations for which they may benefit from outside assistance to formulate a plan of care that differs from their personal beliefs or values (e.g., elective abortion). Examples of outside resources include ethics committee, spiritual advisors and/or clergy, and social services.

Providing care that is both ethical and beneficent is a collaborative effort of the entire surgical team. It is imperative that the perioperative RN, as the patient's moral agent, perform both patient advocacy and moral agency when the patient's ability to act on his or her own behalf is compromised by the effects of anxiety, sedation and anesthesia, and the insult of the surgical experience.

The following is a brief overview of the various regulations, standards, recommended practices, and guidelines that direct professional nursing practice.

- The ANA drafted its first model nurse practice act in 1915; by 1923, all 48 states had enacted nursing licensure laws. Both the state's nurse practice act, and rules and regulations, usually referred to as administrative law, govern the practice of nursing. The legislature of each state is authorized to establish nursing licensure laws that are enforced by the board of nursing. New legislation regarding nurse licensure is usually initiated through the state's nursing association or through the board of nursing at the request of professional nursing organizations. The professional nurse's responsibilities are based on the ANA's *NURSING Scope and Standards of Practice* (ANA, 2004), *Nursing's Social Policy Statement* (ANA, 2003), and *Code of Ethics for Nurses with Interpretive Statements* (ANA, 2001). The nine standards of professional performance, as outlined by the ANA, describe a competent level of behavior in the professional role in the areas of quality of practice, practice evaluation, education, collegiality, collaboration, ethics, research, resource utilization, and leadership (ANA, 2004). The *Code of Ethics for Nurses* (ANA, 2001) provides a structure within which nurses can make ethically sound decisions for patient care, as well as the fulfillment of their responsibilities to the patient, the profession, other members of the care team, and the public.

- AORN develops achievable standards, recommended practices, and guidelines believed to be an optimal level of perioperative nursing practice. Because the practice of perioperative nursing and surgical technology is dynamic, these standards, recommended practices, and guidelines are stated in broad, general terms so they can be adapted to a variety of facilities and practice settings. These standards, recommended practices, and guidelines are based on the most current scientific and theoretical evidence at the time of their development. They are expanded, updated, and revised on a regular basis to reflect current advancements and demands in perioperative nursing and medicine.

- Nursing is also influenced by other guidelines and regulatory agencies. Examples are OSHA, CDC, the American College of Surgeons (ACS), and the American Society of Anesthesiologists (ASA). While OSHA develops both guidelines and regulatory requirements, the CDC, ACS, and ASA develop various guidelines for the care of the patient in surgery that influence the practice of perioperative nursing.

The ever-changing health care environment reinforces the need for all nurses to be knowledgeable of the current regulatory standards, recommended practices, and guidelines applicable to perioperative nursing and the practice of surgery. Compliance with practice standards, recommended practices, and guidelines is critical in ensuring nursing's commitment to society in maintaining accountability and responsibility for the quality of nursing care. Continual education and evaluation of nursing practice, according to the regulations, standards, recommended practices, and guidelines, are vital factors in maintaining the integrity of professional perioperative nursing practice.

Identify and Utilize Resources for Professional Growth

Included in the defining characteristics of a professional is the responsibility to evaluate one's own nursing practice in relation to professional practice standards (e.g., AORN's standards, recommended practices, and guidelines) and relevant state and federal regulations. In so doing, the professional nurse's practice reflects the application of knowledge by providing safe and effective care. There are various methods by which the professional perioperative nurse can demonstrate professional growth (ANA, 2004), such as:

- providing age appropriate care;
- developing a plan of care that incorporates both cultural and ethnic values and wishes of the patient;
- engaging in self-evaluation and developing a plan for professional growth based on the information obtained;
- obtaining peer review regarding one's own practice;
- taking the initiative to achieve goals identified during the self-peer evaluation process;
- implementing changes in practice based on research findings;
- demonstrating one's competency;
- complying with local, state, and federal regulations and accrediting body guidelines;
- practicing according to the ethical codes and standards, recommended practices, and guidelines;
- delegating duties only to competent and appropriate

personnel; and
- intervening to protect patients.

Participate in Quality Improvement Activities

A distinguishing trait of professional nursing is self-regulation for monitoring scope and standards of practice. Nurses regulate themselves through peer review and continuous performance improvement. The registered nurse systematically refines the knowledge, skills, and clinical decision-making processes at all levels and in all areas of nursing by employing performance improvement strategies (ANA, 2003; Griffitts, 2002; ANA, 2004).

The quality improvement process is ingrained within health care systems today and is driven by many national initiatives with reportable quality indicators. The success of any quality improvement process hinges on the participation and support of those directly involved in providing patient care, that being the nurse caring for the patient during surgery. Consequently, the perioperative nurse should understand the basic principles of performance improvement, appreciate his or her role related to specific performance improvement initiatives, and be willing to assume new and different practice patterns to support better patient outcomes.

The performance improvement process requires a commitment from the health care organization, which should be infused throughout the organization and embraced by all providers. Continuous quality improvement is defined as the combination of principles and methods that create both a quality and a patient- and family-centric environment of care, as well as the capability to identify, assess, and constantly enhance the efficiency and effectiveness of those processes that determine significant organizational results. Quality improvement activities are most successful when they involve all staff and when departmental barriers are minimized or eliminated by leadership. The key principles of performance improvement follow.

- Continual improvement is the principal priority of the organization's mission and reflected in daily activities.
- The organization's leaders are committed to and involved in the process (i.e., they drive the process and provide the necessary resources and also remove or at least minimize barriers to success).
- The primary focus is on the functions that influence outcomes; it is necessary to improve work processes and systems that support quality patient care, not just solve crises.
- Data are available, meaningful, and used in the decision-making process, including feedback from patients and other providers. In addition, the information system should support ease of data entry, collection, retrieval, and analysis.
- All staff members are responsible individually and collectively for the performance improvement process by actualizing autonomy in the performance of their role, reducing internal barriers, and supporting a multi-disciplinary improvement process.

There are various quality improvement activities that the perioperative RN can participate in. Such activities may include:

- identifying aspects of practice important for quality monitoring (e.g., maintaining normothermia during the intraoperative period);
- using indicators suggested by professional nursing or other organizations to monitor quality and effectiveness of nursing practice (e.g., PNDS Outcome Indicators [Beyea, 2002]);
- collecting data to monitor the quality and effectiveness of nursing practice;
- analyzing data to identify opportunities for improvement;
- devising recommendations to improve nursing practice and outcomes;
- implementing activities to improve the quality of care provided to patients;
- reviewing, developing, implementing, and evaluating organizational policies and procedures;
- participating on committees or interdisciplinary teams evaluating clinical care or health care services or systems of care delivery;
- participating in cost-containment activities; and
- analyzing incident reports and learning from past experiences.

In today's dynamic health care environment, ensuring quality patient care and satisfaction, as well as implementing performance improvement measures are key elements in the delivery of cost-effective, efficient care. The perioperative nurse has an ethical and professional obligation to be knowledgable of and participate in both departmental and organizational performance improvement activities. The perioperative nurse should understand the principles of quality and performance improvement, data collection, and analysis methods, and also actively participate in the process by providing input and feedback.

Perioperative nurses, by virtue of their professional obligation, are obliged to advance the knowledge and skills of nursing practice by engaging in activities that enlarge, disseminate, and implement research findings. Use of the PNDS is one way that perioperative nurses may participate in research and promote evidence-based practice. The PNDS provides data elements (i.e., quality indicators) linked to specific patient outcomes that are codified and operationally defined in such a way to provide the foundation for gathering data about the effect of nursing care during the perioperative experience.

Perioperative nurses can participate in research as content experts, by asking "why we do it that way" and conducting a systematic review of the literature to determine what is supported by research, by participating in research projects, or by conducting research. Perioperative nurses have a professional responsibility individually and collectively for advancing the profession through active involvement in self-regulation by participating in peer review, quality improvement, and evidence-based practice.

Summary

Establishing and maintaining professional accountability are essential to the professionalism of the nurse. The key characteristics of professional accountability in nursing are:

- lifelong learning, continual knowledge and skill acquisition, and annual competency validation;
- incorporating regulations and professional practice standards, recommended practices, and guidelines into daily practice;
- supporting the professional growth of self, peers, colleagues, and other health care professionals;
- participating in and evaluating performance improvement activities;
- incorporating the *Code of Ethics for Nurses* (ANA, 2001) and AORN's Explications for Perioperative Nursing (AORN, 2006) into daily practice;
- developing and enhancing critical thinking and problem solving skills;
- developing and participating in collaborative (e.g., multidisciplinary committee or work groups) perioperative practice; and
- incorporating (nursing) research findings and/or conducting research to expand the knowledge base and practice of perioperative nursing.

There are many ways to demonstrate professional accountability in nursing practice. One of the ways to demonstrate one's accountability as a professional perioperative nurse is through certification (e.g., CNOR, CRNFA). Successful completion of the certification process is evidence of an increased level of knowledge, skill, and competence as a perioperative professional nurse. In today's dynamic perioperative environment and diversity of practice settings, the perioperative nurse should continually update and maintain the requisite knowledge and skills as a competent care provider if one is to meet his or her individual professional responsibilities to patients, the profession, and society.

Case Studies/Discussion Points

Case Study 1

JJ, a CNOR-certified registered nurse from an agency, is assigned to the scrub role in your room. You are setting up for a laparoscopic-assisted vaginal hysterectomy (LAVH). While you and JJ are setting up the room, you notice that she has brightly-colored artificial nails, is wearing a lovely pearl necklace over her scrub top, and has matching long dangling earrings hanging outside her scrub cap. You know that this is against AORN's Recommended Practices for Surgical Attire and a violation of your facility's policy and procedure for surgical attire. You approach JJ to explain her violation with AORN's recommended practices and facility policy and procedure for surgical attire.

Discussion Points for Case Study 1

1. What knowledge is JJ lacking in regards to proper surgical attire?
2. Has anyone reviewed or oriented her to your policy and procedure?
3. What professional recommended practices and guidelines (e.g., AORN, CDC, OSHA, and Association for Professionals in Infection Control) outline appropriate surgical attire?
4. Is there evidence to support the recommendation concerning the wearing of artificial nails, nail polish, and/or jewelry in the patient care setting?
5. What is the potential impact on patient outcomes, if any?

Responses to consider:

1. What knowledge is JJ lacking in regards to proper surgical attire?

- JJ is lacking knowledge of AORN's Recommended Practices for Surgical Attire which state: "All personnel entering the semi restricted and restricted areas of the surgical suite should confine or remove all jewelry and watches. Artificial nails should not be worn" (AORN, 2006).

2. Is there any scientific evidence supporting these recommended practices?

- Yes, AORN recommended practices are based on research studies that support the practices that have been recommended. Arrowsmith and colleagues (2004) and Trick, et al (2003) found that rings, watches, and bracelets harbor organisms that cannot be removed during hand washing. Another study looking at artificial nails (Moolenarr, et al, 2000) found that fungal growth occurs frequently under artificial nails as a result of moisture trapped between the artificial nail and natural nail. This study identified the wearing of artificial nails as the cause of a prolonged outbreak of *Pseudomonas aeruginosa* in a neonatal intensive care unit.

3. How might JJ's attire affect patient outcomes?

- There are strong experimental, clinical, and epidemiological studies and theoretical rationale supporting an increase in the risk of postoperative surgical site infection when recommended practices for surgical attire are not followed (CDC, 1999).

- Using recommended practices and guidelines for guidance in developing facility policy and procedure and incorporating them into your daily clinical practice is a means of creating evidence-based practice.

Case Study 2

RS, a certified registered nurse anesthetist has been practicing as an anesthesia care provider for eight years in the same hospital. RS has always been very conscientious in his practice (e.g., conducting thorough preoperative patient interviews, setting up his equipment early, collaborating with all members of the surgical team). During the past six months, you and other staff have noticed a change in RS's behavior: he frequently comes to work "just-in-time," and even late on some occasions; he has become increasingly impatient with both patients and coworkers; and sometimes appears distracted during longer cases. In addition, the postanesthesia care unit (PACU) nurses are reporting that RS's patients usually are requiring more pain medication than in the past. Today, you are assigned to a right hemicolectomy and RS is the anesthesia care provider. Midway through the case, you see RS has his head down on the anesthesia machine and by all appearances is asleep.

Discussion Points for Case Study 2

1. What is the risk to the patient?
2. Whom must you advocate for and protect in this situation?
3. What is your professional and ethical obligation in this situation?

Responses to consider:

1. What is the risk to the patient?

- The most obvious risk is the potential for harm to the patient because the provider appears to be impaired and may not able to optimally perform the duties of his role.

2. Whom must you advocate for and protect in this situation?

- In this situation you have a dual responsibility. First and foremost you must take action to protect the patient from harm. It is imperative to notify your charge nurse and the supervising anesthesiologist of the situation so that patient care will not be compromised. You also have an obligation to RS in reporting the situation to his supervisor so that he may evaluate and receive the appropriate intervention or refusals for assistance.

3. What is your professional and ethical obligation in this situation?

- The potential risk of harm to the patient must be removed. You have a professional and ethical obligation to report your observations immediately to the anesthesiologist supervising RS for intercession to protect the patient. You also should report the situation to your manager following your facility chain of command, as the situation has facility wide ramifications. The anesthesiologist is responsible for taking action to protect the patient by removing RS from the case and replacing him with a capable anesthesia care provider. Perioperative nurses should be aware of the various programs and resources available to health care providers affected by mental and physical illness or by personal circumstances (e.g., substance abuse, addiction) that impair their ability to perform the duties of their job.

Suggested Learning Activities

As a continuation of the self-assessment process, the following activities may be helpful in increasing your level of expertise regarding establishing and maintaining professional accountability as a perioperative nurse:

- Review your state nurse practice act. This document will outline the legal definitions and scope of practice in your state. Also review OSHA, JCAHO, and CDC recommendations and guidelines that relate to the operative and invasive procedure.

- Review the ANA's *Code of Ethics for Nurses* (ANA, 2001) and AORN's Explications for Perioperative Nursing. AORN offers a self-directed learning module, Ethics in Perioperative Practice (AORN, 2004) that will help perioperative nurses relate the ANA's *Code of Ethics for Nurses with Interpretive Statements* to their own areas of practice.

- Review AORN's current *Standards, Recommended Practices, and Guidelines*, paying particular attention to those areas that are new or newly revised, and those areas in which you may need further knowledge and skill acquisition.

- Read monthly professional journals and focus on research article(s) and home studies. Begin or participate in an existing journal club that looks at a clinical practice article and critiques the study findings for application to nursing practice.

- Volunteer to be a member of your OR's performance improvement committee to gain a better understanding of the quality improvement process and how you can contribute to improving patient care. Examine your practice to identify practice issues and review the literature/evidence as to what is considered best practice and/or a cost-effective method of performing a specific intervention or activity.

- Describe an area in your practice in which you can help a colleague or coworker increase his or her knowledge. Be a preceptor to new employees, nursing interns, and/or nursing and allied health professional students. Develop an individual orientation or education process to provide education and training to your colleagues, and then solicit your colleague's feedback on your effectiveness. This could be as simple as teaching your coworkers how to use a new piece of equipment (e.g., in-service activities).

- Challenge yourself to increase your knowledge and critical thinking skills.

- Collaborate with your coworker on issues, especially on conflict situations. Think of the elements of collaboration, communication, accountability, competency, respect for personhood, and trust.

- Discuss ethical issues in the perioperative environment (e.g., cost containment, organ donation, do-not-resuscitate) with your coworkers and your facility ethics committee. Discuss how the perioperative nurse can assist the patient and family facing ethical issues or decision making concerning health care directives.

Chapter 10

Strategies for Success: Getting Prepared and Being Test-Wise

Linda D. Waters, RN, PhD

Being successful at passing the CNOR certification examination for perioperative nursing requires having a thorough and sound foundation of the knowledge and skills required for expert clinical practice as well as an understanding of the test-taking process. Knowledge is attained through both work experiences and formal educational programs. The experiential knowledge component requires that an individual who is eligible to take the CNOR certification examination have a minimum of two years of work experience in perioperative nursing. The knowledge component is acquired through a variety of learning activities, including formal education, self-study, and continuing education programs, all aiming to promote continuing competency. It is the combination of experiential and cognitive knowledge that forms the foundation of expert clinical practice.

In addition to this evidenced-based clinical knowledge, you will also need to have a firm understanding of the testing process. Being familiar with the testing process will not only prepare you to take the test but will also acquaint you with the environment in which the test will be given. There is a definite skill in answering multiple-choice test questions. Becoming familiar with these techniques will improve your chances of successful performance on the CNOR certification examination.

This chapter provides information about planning your personalized study program, obtaining the necessary resources to assist in your preparation, understanding the processes involved with answering multiple-choice test questions, and developing sound test-taking strategies to lead to success on your CNOR certification examination.

Learning Objectives

Upon completion of this chapter, the individual should be able to:

1. Identify specific content areas in perioperative nursing where you will need further knowledge.

2. Develop an action plan for acquiring additional knowledge in content areas where needed.

3. Identify resources that will be of assistance in preparing for the CNOR certification examination.

4. Identify the major components of multiple-choice test questions.

5. Develop skill in applying test-taking strategies when answering multiple-choice test questions.

6. Plan a success-oriented action plan for taking the CNOR certification examination.

Developing Good Study Habits

Making the initial decision to take a certification examination is an important decision. For most test takers, becoming certified in a specialty area of nursing practice accomplishes both personal and professional goals. The personal goal is a feeling of accomplishment—tackling a task that may be difficult yet, at the same time, rewarding. Professionally, certification provides external recognition of excellence in nursing and may promote career advancements. In addition, certification is a symbol of achievement that distinguishes the credential holder from others in the field. The certificate holder can proudly state that he or she has met a standard of achievement established by experts in nursing.

The next step in the certification process is determining what your personal investment will be in preparing for the examination. And, what a personal investment it is! The easiest part is paying the examination fee. The more difficult part is determining realistically what you want to do and can do to prepare for the examination. Each person will need to decide what works best for them. Ultimately, when you go to your testing appointment, you want to be certain you are as prepared as you can be and are confident about your ability to demonstrate your command of perioperative nursing knowledge.

Use the following questions to determine what your personal investment in your preparation for your certification examination will be.

Question #1 — Should I Study for the Examination?

Studying for the examination is your choice and is, in no small way, a decision based on your years of experience in perioperative nursing. While experience is critical, your personal work experiences may not have provided you with the broad skills and knowledge needed to be successful on the certification examination. Remember, a certification examination is a general examination that will ask questions about many areas of perioperative nursing. Ask yourself whether your experiences in perioperative nursing have been sufficiently broad enough to prepare you for all content areas that might be included on the test. Are there areas of practice with which you have not had work experience or where standards of practice may have recently changed?

So, do you need to study? Conduct a self-assessment to determine your chances for passing the certification examination. How do you do that?

An excellent starting point is to review critical documents, including the *CNOR Test Blueprint* and the current AORN *Standards, Recommended Practices, and Guidelines.* For each content area that is identified, assess your "level of competency." Conduct this assessment before you register and schedule your examination to allow sufficient preparation time before the examination. Use a rating scale such as the one below to determine what you believe to be your current level of competency.

> 1—*Very Certain:* I know this content area well and believe that my work experiences have fully prepared me. I am comfortable with current practices and believe I am up-to-date with new developments and advances.
>
> 2—*Certain:* I am reasonably comfortable with this content area and believe that my work experiences have prepared me fairly well.
>
> 3—*Undecided:* I have some knowledge and some experiences in this area, but there may be a few content areas where I am not as strong or for which my work experiences have not fully prepared me.
>
> 4—*Uncertain:* I am aware that I have some knowledge deficits and/or a lack of work experience in this content area. I will need to engage in some study or other remediation to be comfortable with this content area.
>
> 5—*Very Uncertain:* I am aware that I have many knowledge deficits and/or lack work experiences in this content area. This is an area of weakness for me and one which will require me to remediate before taking the examination.

Then apply this rating scale to each area of the *CNOR Test Blueprint.* Be completely honest with your self-assessment—remember, it is intended to help you prepare for the CNOR examination. If you rate all areas as 1 or 2, you may find that you will need little to no preparation before taking the examination. If, on the other hand, you find that you have a mixture of responses, rating some 1 and 2 and other 3, 4, or 5, you may find it very useful to develop an individualized study plan that will allow you sufficient time to prepare before taking the examination.

Knowing that you have done all you can to prepare for taking the CNOR certification examination will give you that extra boost of confidence! And, it also will help you determine when to schedule your examination within the testing period.

Be realistic! Preparing for the examination will be best completed over a period of weeks, not days or hours. Don't shortchange yourself. Allow sufficient study time before the examination.

Question #2 — What Should I Study?

Go back to the self-assessment you completed when making the decision whether to study. Consider dividing the content areas from the *CNOR Test Blueprint* into three broad areas:

> Area 1—Content that I have knowledge strengths.
>
> Area 2—Content that is mixed—I may know some areas but have weaknesses in others.
>
> Area 3—Content that I know I have knowledge weaknesses.

Then look at the proportion of the test that is dedicated to each area you identified. Concentrate your study time on those areas of the *CNOR Test Blueprint* where you have the greatest knowledge weaknesses and where the largest percentage of test questions will be represented. Tackle those needs *FIRST*, before going on to other areas.

Question #3 — What is the Best Study Style for Me?

Once you have decided that you do want to study for the examination and you have developed a study plan specific to your needs, next determine a study style that works best for you. Remember back to your school days. What worked best for you then? Were you more successful when you studied alone in the privacy of your own study space? Or, were you more focused when you studied with others? Maybe a combination study style works best for you—individual study for reviewing familiar concepts and group study for learning new content areas.

What will likely be different now from your earlier study experiences in high school or college is the amount of time you have available for study. Looking back, those earlier days were a lot easier when you had fewer commitments. As you prepare for your certification examination you must balance your other commitments (e.g., family, work) with your need to prepare for the examination.

Plan the best time for taking the examination. If you know that the next few months are especially busy for you with unusual work expectations (e.g., staff shortages, preparing for an accreditation visit) or family responsibilities (e.g., vacation, childcare, holidays), don't add to these burdens by scheduling the examination during that period. Remember, you have the flexibility to choose a testing time that works best for you. Because the CNOR certification examination is available on a daily basis throughout the year, register and schedule the examination at a time that is best for you—a time that allows you adequate preparation and no other major commitments or conflicts.

Remember, this certification examination is important for you both personally and professionally. Once you have made the commitment to take the examination, commit also to developing a personalized study plan—and stick to it! Engage help from your family, friends, and colleagues to stick to your study plan.

Question #4 — How Do I Plan and Manage My Study Time

Once you have completed your self-assessment and identified what you need to study, you will be able to develop a study schedule that, if adhered to, should guide you to a successful testing experience. Obviously, the more knowledge weaknesses you identify in major areas that will be covered on the CNOR certification examination, the greater time you will need to allow for fulfilling your study schedule.

Most important is to stay focused and committed to your study plan. You will be most confident if you plan for your study time and stick to the study schedule you develop. Use your study time wisely. Make use of any spare time that you have to review concepts.

Here are some suggestions to make the best use of your study time.

- Consider making flashcards out of index cards and carry those with you everywhere. That way even an extra five minutes can be turned into valuable study time.

- Develop a note-taking system from your study periods. That way you will have a record of what areas you have reviewed and areas still outstanding.

- Organize your notes according to their importance for the content area on the examination. In that way, if you have only a short amount of time to study one day, you can go right to the notes of greatest importance.

- Make a practice of learning about one new fact at each study session.

- Use your work experiences as an avenue for study. Be certain to learn about new procedures, new therapies, and other developments that you encounter in your day-to-day work experiences. Seek out new learning opportunities.

Question #5 — What Do I Study?

There are many excellent sources for study materials. Most importantly, be sure to review important AORN documents. The *AORN Journal* is an excellent resource for the latest knowledge in perioperative nursing. Because the timelines for printing journals are much shorter than textbooks, be sure to use journals as the source for new developments and important changes in perioperative nursing practice.

A second important source for review will be the "classic" textbooks in perioperative nursing. Look to see what textbooks are frequently cited in the literature or are the textbooks that everyone refers to when questions arise. Plan to spend some time reviewing these books. As you prepare for the CNOR certification examination, let these be your "best sellers."

Look to technology to provide a third source of study materials. There are excellent resources that can be found through the Internet. Consider combining your study preparation with earning continuing education units. Complete continuing education programs that can be found on-line, or simply call up a topic of interest and search the Internet to see what is available.

Handy Study Tips

- *Study everyday—even if the best you can mange is a few minutes.* Studying every day helps you to stick with your commitment to prepare for the examination, will help you feel a sense of accomplishment, and will help avoid "last minute panic."

- *Balance "old" learning with "new" learning.* As you prepare for the examination, you will find some content areas where you need to simply review or "brush up" on your knowledge. In other cases, you may discover "new" content areas that you will need to learn. Remember that the examination is a general examination in perioperative nursing and the content areas evaluated by the examination may include areas in which you have not previously worked. Try to balance your study sessions to allow some new knowledge gains along with the review of more familiar content.

- *Use your work setting as your personal learning center.* In some ways, each workday provides you with an excellent opportunity to prepare for the examination. See how you can build in new knowledge in your daily activities. For example, are you administering a drug that is not used frequently? Use that opportunity to go to a reference and learn more about the drug. Are you assisting in a surgical procedure? Ask questions of your colleagues and find out all you can, especially about areas that are less familiar to you.

- *Let your work colleagues know that you are preparing for your certification examination.* Sharing your plans to take the certification examination with your work colleagues will accomplish two purposes. First, ask them to "remind" you that you need to prepare for the examination. Your colleagues can be a great source of support and encouragement. Give them the "okay" to ask you if you are on schedule with your preparation. Second, ask your colleagues to become your study coaches. Remind them to seek you out when they have an interesting surgical case or when there is a new learning opportunity. You may want to share with your colleagues the areas where you believe you have knowledge weaknesses so they can be on the alert for study opportunities that relate.

- *Stay focused on your goal.* At some point in your study cycle, you will no doubt ask yourself, "Why did I decide to do this?" It is normal to feel a bit overwhelmed, but sticking to your goal will be rewarding.

Components of a Multiple-Choice Test Question

In addition to a planned study program, you should work to develop your knowledge and skill in answering multiple-choice questions. It is important that you understand the structure and format of this type of test question.

Experts in perioperative nursing write the questions for the CNOR certification examination. As such, each question is written to assess important knowledge and skills essential for competent perioperative nursing practice. Much effort goes into developing each question, including multiple reviews by many subject matter experts. Questions are never designed to "trick" the test taker.

Each question on the examination is a four-option, multiple-choice test question (or item). A multiple-choice test question consists of the stem and the options. The stem provides the information that supports the question that is being asked. It should contain sufficient information for you to understand what is being asked, even by just reading it alone.

The stem is followed by four options, one of which is the correct answer (or key) as determined by a panel of content experts and documented by current literature. The other three options are the distracters, which are plausible but not correct answers. There is one and only one best answer among the options provided.

The stem of each test question may be closed-ended or open-ended. A closed-ended question asks a complete question and ends with a question mark. An open-ended question is a type of fill-in-the-blank with the four choices provided as the options. Each of the choices will complete the statement.

The following are examples of each question format:

Closed-ended question:

- Which of the following is the rationale for having perioperative nursing personnel immunized with hepatitis B vaccine?
  1. Current legislation requires the immunization.
  2. Occupational risk of acquiring the hepatitis virus is high.*
  3. The immunization also provides protection against other forms of hepatitis.
  4. Standard precautions require routine immunization for all bloodborne viruses.

Open-ended question:

- Perioperative nursing personnel should receive hepatitis B immunization because:
  1. current legislation requires the immunization.
  2. the occupational risk of acquiring the hepatitis virus is high.*
  3. the immunization also provides protection against other forms of hepatitis.
  4. standard precautions require routine immunization for all bloodborne viruses.

The multiple-choice test questions used in the CNOR certification examination measure either basic knowledge or pose a situation where an application of the knowledge is required. Because clinical practice requires the ability to apply principles and facts to patient situations, most of the test questions on the CNOR certification examination are at the application level. The following are examples of these two types of questions:

Knowledge/Comprehension:

- The loss of heat from exposed body parts due to exposure of air currents is known as:
  1. evaporation.
  2. conduction.
  3. radiation.
  4. convection.*

Application:

- During skin preparation, the scrub person informs the perioperative nurse that the sleeve of a student's warm-up jacket has brushed against the area being prepared. Which of the following would be an appropriate response for the perioperative nurse to take *first*?
  1. Report the incident to the instructor for followup.
  2. Have the student review the required technique.
  3. Review skin preparation at the next inservice program.
  4. Inform the student immediately of the break in technique.*

Before any question is added to the CNOR certification examination, it is "pretested" on a representative group of test takers to ensure that the question performs statistically as intended. This occurs before the question is included and scored in an actual test administration.

One point is given for each correct answer. The total score on the examination is the total points given for all correct answers. There is no penalty for guessing so answer all questions. Budget your time wisely to complete the entire test.

Taking the CNOR Certification Examination

The CNOR certification examination is a computer-based test that is administered at a test center. Each testing candidate schedules an individualized testing appointment for a date and time that is convenient for them. Unlike paper-and-pencil tests where there may be several hundred individuals in the same room, the test center is designed to accommodate about 10 to 15 computer stations and each person in the testing room may be taking a different examination. Some of these examinations may be shorter or longer than the CNOR certification examination, so you will notice that others either are leaving the room ahead of you or are still taking their examination when you have finished.

When the examination begins, you will first be given a brief on-screen tutorial that will orient you to taking a test on a computer. Remember that you do not need computer skills or familiarity with a computer to take the CNOR certification examination. And, even if you are very skilled in using a computer, the tutorial that is part of the examination will teach you how to navigate within this examination.

While the mouse is more commonly used, the keyboard is enabled for use in answering questions. In addition, the tutorial will provide instructions on using the various features: "Previous," which allows you to return to a previously seen question; "Mark," which allows you to identify specific test questions that you would like to return to at a later time whether you have answered the question or skipped it; and "Review," which presents a list of all of the test questions and highlights those questions that you have marked. As you proceed through the test, you may skip a question and return to it later to answer. You may review questions at any time, not only at the end of the test.

You should complete the tutorial in its entirety, focusing on how the features of the test operate so that you are familiar with these functions. Your answers to the practice questions in the tutorial are not included in your test score.

The test center staff that proctors the examination and monitors your activities will be located in the room outside the testing room and are available if you need assistance. They are not content experts about perioperative nursing, so they are not able to provide you with any assistance about the test questions themselves. Their role is to monitor the activities in the testing room and report any unusual situations or inappropriate behavior. If you have a concern about a test question, you will have an opportunity to report your concern at the end of the examination.

You will find more information about the testing situation in the *CNOR Certification Recertification Policy Manual.* In addition, your *Authorization to Test* (ATT) that will be mailed to you includes instructions about the day of the examination, what time to arrive at the testing center, what identification you will need, and other general guidelines.

How to Take Tests

For many individuals, the CNOR certification examination will be the first test taken in many years. The mere thought of sitting for four hours answering multiple-choice questions brings back memories of earlier testing situations. So it is important that you prepare yourself to be in the best physical and mental condition that is possible.

Keep yourself in good physical health before the examination date. You should plan to eat a balanced meal the evening before and then get a good night's sleep. Plan to eat breakfast before a morning appointment (or lunch before an afternoon appointment), because you will be in the testing room for over four hours. Avoid over-eating though, as too much food or liquids could make you tired. Feeling well and being rested are important strategies for success. You need to be able to read carefully and think clearly.

Some people become anxious about the testing situation and have difficulty focusing and processing complex information. Mental anxiety stimulates the stress hormones, which have a direct impact on the cerebral cortex resulting in a decreased ability to think clearly and problem solve. When this happens, you can become irritable and restless, be unable to sleep, and have difficulty thinking.

One way to reduce this anxiety is to desensitize yourself to a potentially stressful situation. You can accomplish this by preparing for the examination, taking several practice tests, and developing a sense of calm about the situation. As you feel better prepared, you will find that you can become less anxious.

Test-Taking Guidelines

Being successful in passing the certification examination takes more than just knowing the content. You need to understand how to read and answer multiple-choice test questions. There is a very simple and easy-to-follow strategy in taking multiple-choice tests.

When reading multiple-choice test questions, it is important to remember that there is one and only one correct answer. So, consider the following.

- *Attempt to answer the question before reading the options and then look for an option that best fits your answer.* You should be able to answer a good multiple-choice question without reading the options. Cover up the options and see if you can determine an answer to the question being asked. Then, uncover the options. Often you will find that your answer is one of the options provided. In that case, your best course of action is to go with your first answer. Try to avoid changing an answer.

- *Note that the options are written to be plausible to those who do not know the content.* Well-written multiple-choice questions are designed to have four plausible options. The intent is to discriminate between those candidates who know the information and those who do not. If you are unsure of the answer, try to eliminate options that you believe are incorrect. This improves your chance of selecting the correct answer.

- *Eliminate options that have absolutes, such as "always" or "never."* There is very little in nursing practice that is absolute. Most courses of action in clinical practice and most client responses are "usually" or "generally."

- *Read the question carefully, paying special attention to phrases, such as "most," "most appropriate," "primarily," "first," and "initially."* Often all of the options are applicable to the situation, but only one option fits the emphasis included in the stem.

- *Take careful note of words such as "not," "least," or "except."* These words in the stem tend to confuse the reader, because the correct answer for the test question is the wrong response or the wrong thing to do.

- *Answer all of the questions.* Credit is given for all correct answers. So if you are unsure of an answer, take an educated guess among the plausible options.

- *Monitor your progress by noting the time remaining on the computer screen.* The CNOR certification examination is timed to provide you with about one minute per question. If you find that you are taking more time than expected to answer a question, mark the question and return to it once you have finished reading through the entire test. You do not want to spend too much time reading one test question and then run out of time, leaving several questions at the end unanswered. Unanswered questions will be scored as incorrect.

- *Review your work after you have completed the test.* Once you have read through the test and answered as many questions as you can, you should return to review the questions that you may have skipped or marked for further review. Then, if there is available time when you have completed the entire test, you can review all of the questions and reconsider your choices. You should refrain from making too many changes. Often, test takers change a right response to a wrong response.

How to Avoid Making Errors

Being successful in passing the certification examination requires that you also avoid making mistakes in answering the test questions. One helpful strategy to avoid test-taking errors is to take practice tests. Become familiar with the format of multiple-choice questions. Use the CNOR practice tests as a method of improving your knowledge and identifying areas for further study.

When answering practice questions, consider the following as methods to avoid making testing errors:

- *Read each question carefully.* Errors are made when you do not read the question carefully. Look for and identify the important points involved with the question. Read each option carefully, noting which option most closely matches the intent of the question. Eliminate the options that are not plausible.

- *Assume that all of the information you need is presented in the test question.* The stem of a multiple-choice test question should contain all of the information that is necessary for the test taker to answer the question. When you read the question, avoid the common pitfall of "reading into" the question. Doing this may only confuse you. If certain patient characteristics, such as age, diagnosis, clinical setting, or other related information, are important to know to answer the question, it is provided. Otherwise, answer the question from the perspective of the most common situation.

- *Identify content areas where your knowledge base is weak.* Use the practice test as an opportunity to evaluate your current knowledge of perioperative nursing. When you answer questions incorrectly, use the opportunity to learn the reasons for the incorrect answers. Ask yourself, "Why was my choice wrong?" The best way to learn the content is to understand the underlying rationale for the correct as well as the incorrect answers.

- *Understand the basic intent of the test question.* One of the most common errors that test takers make is not understanding the intent of the question. Is the question asking for you to make a decision about identifying a priority, a sequence of events, or an important patient presentation? Often in these types of questions, all of the options are plausible for the situation, but the correct answer is the one that is most important, has the highest priority, or is the first action to be taken. Look for the guiding words that give you the direction or emphasis to take.

Day-of-Test Checklist

Within 24 hours before the examination, you should:

- *Avoid engaging in any known stressful events.* Many of us know what events tend to cause us stress. If at all possible, try to avoid engaging in or attending events that are known stressors just before taking the examination. Practice using relaxation methods to create a calm mental perspective about the test. This will minimize the production of stress hormones and enable you to think clearly and problem solve the questions.

- *Obtain sufficient rest and sleep.* Fatigue and lethargy will only inhibit your thinking and problem-solving abilities. Engage in any sleep rituals that tend to promote your sleeping ability.

- *Limit use of any stimulants, including coffee.* Stimulants will affect your ability to receive sufficient rest and sleep. Avoid taking any stimulants, including coffee, late in the day and before bedtime the night before the test.

- *Review the CNOR confirmation packet with regard to your responsibilities on the day of the examination.* It is your responsibility to be aware of the rules and regulations regarding the CNOR testing experience. If you do not follow the rules as outlined in the confirmation packet, you can be denied access to the testing center. After all of your studying and planning, you do not want to forfeit your testing opportunity at the last minute.

- *Arrive at the testing center at least 30 minutes before your test appointment.* If you are unsure of the exact location of the test center, it is strongly suggested that you locate the test center ahead of time. Determine how long it will take you to drive there or go by public transportation, if applicable, by following the route before the day of your test. The test center can provide you with directions if you need them or go online and print out directions. Unforeseen and uncontrollable events, such as accidents or inclement weather, can cause delays in your travel time. It is far better to be early than to be late and miss your appointment.

- *Bring few personal items with you.* Limit the personal items you bring with you. You will not be permitted to take handbags, wallets, books, cellular phones, laptops, or any other personal belongings into the testing room. The test center has lockers where you can store any items you bring. The proctor will provide you with scrap paper. There is no space at the test center for family members or friends to accompany you to your testing appointment.

- *Make sure that you bring the following items with you to the test center:*
  - Authorization to Test. This letter informs the test center staff of your eligibility to test, your name, and the test that you are taking.
  - Two forms of identification, one of which must be a current, government-issued photo identification, such as a driver's license or a passport, with a signature. Be sure your identification matches exactly the name on your Authorization to Test.
  - Watch.

After the Exam

- *Try to avoid "second guessing."* While it is common practice to "relive" the test experience, try not to second guess the responses you gave to each test question. Without the content of the question directly in front of you, it is too easy to "conclude" you may have answered incorrectly.

- *Do not share information about the test or test questions.* Remember that you have signed a pledge to keep the contents of the CNOR certification examination confidential. Sharing information about the test or discussing specific questions about the test with colleagues or other test takers violates this confidentiality pledge. In addition, multiple forms of the examination are being administered so it is highly likely that the questions you saw on your test will not be the exact same questions another test taker saw.

Summary

Being successful occurs when you have made a detailed plan for preparing for the examination and stick to it! Identifying knowledge areas for review, taking frequent practice tests, understanding the testing process, and getting yourself into the best mental state are essential components of success.

Suggested Learning Activities

As part of your action plan for success, you may consider some of the following learning activities helpful.

- Develop a reference list of textbooks, journals, and on-line educational opportunities that will provide you with the necessary information to expand your knowledge base of perioperative nursing.

- Begin studying those areas that you have identified as being your weak areas.

- Organize a study group of coworkers and other colleagues, if possible.

- Attend as many continuing education programs that are available.

- Practice taking multiple-choice test questions by answering the questions in Appendix I of this book.

- Commit yourself to a study plan and stick to it.

Appendix I

Practice Questions

1. A patient who is scheduled for arthroscopy of the left knee states that the surgery is for the repair of a torn cartilage in the right knee. The surgical consent form indicates the left knee. The nurse's best action is to:
   A. delay surgery until patient information and consent are validated.
   B. proceed as scheduled, since the patient has signed the consent form.
   C. document the conflict on the OR nursing-care record.
   D. change the consent form and have the patient initial the change.

   Reference: *Berry and Kohn's Operating Room Technique,* Phillips, N., 10th ed., 2004, pages 33-34.

2. The primary concern of the perioperative nurse when evaluating and selecting new medical devices and products for use in the perioperative practice setting is:
   A. cost/value analysis.
   B. ease of use.
   C. patient safety.
   D. environmental impact.

   Reference: *Standards, Recommended Practices and Guidelines,* AORN, Inc., 2006, page 593.

3. During a surgical procedure involving the use of an electrosurgery unit, the surgeon requests an increase in the power setting. The perioperative nurse's first response would be to:
   A. check the ESU circuit beginning with the dispersive electrode.
   B. confirm the increased power setting with the surgeon.
   C. replace the unit with another ESU.
   D. check for incompatibility of the active electrode.

   Reference: *Standards, Recommended Practices and Guidelines,* AORN, Inc., 2006, page 483.

4. Potential adverse effects of the supine position include all of the following except:
   A. skin breakdown at heels and elbows.
   B. venous pooling in the legs.
   C. decreased mean arterial pressure.
   D. retinal detachment or cerebral edema.

   Reference: *Alexander's Care of the Patient in Surgery,* Rothrock, J.C., 12th ed, 2003, page 176.

5. Wearing cover apparel outside the perioperative setting is:
   A. effective in reducing surgical wound infections.
   B. determined by the individual practice setting.
   C. required by OSHA and other regulatory agencies.
   D. considered part of personal protective equipment.

   Reference: *Standards, Recommended Practices and Guidelines,* AORN, Inc., 2006, page 452.

6. Surgical procedures performed on the alimentary, respiratory, or genitourinary tracts without spillage are classified as:
   A. clean.
   B. clean - contaminated.
   C. contaminated.
   D. dirty.

   Reference: *Berry and Kohn's Operating Room Technique,* Phillips, N., 10th ed., 2004, page 568.

7. According to the American Society of Anesthesiologists (ASA) physical status classification, it would be appropriate for a perioperative nurse to monitor a patient classified as a:
   A. P2
   B. P3
   C. P4
   D. P5

   Reference: *Standards, Recommended Practices and Guidelines,* AORN, Inc., 2006, pages 435-436.

8. The herniorrhaphy surgical procedure that involves repairing the defect in the transversalis fascia below the inguinal ligament is known as:
   A. umbilical.
   B. femoral.

C. hiatal.
D. ventral.

Reference: *Berry and Kohn's Operating Room Technique,* Phillips, N., 10th ed., 2004, page 668.

9. According to the AORN recommended practices, an effective surgical hand antisepsis/hand scrub with specific products is effective with a scrub time of how many minutes?
A. 1 to 2
B. 2 to 3
C. 3 to 4
D. 4 to 5

Reference: *Standards, Recommended Practices and Guidelines,* AORN, Inc., 2006, page 542.

10. An instrument used to cut into the bone is called:
A. elevator.
B. rongeur.
C. clamp.
D. curette.

Reference: *Berry and Kohn's Operating Room Technique,* Phillips, N., 10th ed., 2004, page 745.

11. During the preoperative assessment, it is noted that the patient has periods of dyspnea while lying flat. During transport to the operating room, the most appropriate intervention would be to:
A. complete the transport quickly.
B. elevate the head of the transportation vehicle.
C. instruct the holding room nurse to accompany the patient.
D. order portable O_2 for the patient.

Reference: *Alexander's Care of the Patient in Surgery,* Rothrock, J.C., 12th ed, 2003, page 169.

12. The process of cataract removal in which the cataract is broken up by ultrasonic vibration and then aspirated is termed:
A. cryoextractor.
B. diathermy coagulation.
C. laser therapy.
D. phacoemulsification.

Reference: *Berry and Kohn's Operating Room Technique,* Phillips, N., 10th ed., 2004, pages 803-806.

13. Reusable tourniquet cuffs that have come in contact with blood, should be cleaned between patient use according to the manufacturer's instructions by which of the following methods?
A. steam sterilization.
B. high level disinfection.
C. low level disinfection.
D. ethylene oxide sterilization.

Reference: *Standards, Recommended Practices and Guidelines,* AORN, Inc., 2006, pages 469-470.

14. Patient information necessary for accurate arterial blood gas value determination includes the:
A. percentage of oxygen administered and the oxygen flow rate.
B. incision time and the clamping of blood vessels.
C. use of heparin and vitamin K.
D. type of intravenous fluids and the transfusion of blood.

Reference: *Berry and Kohn's Operating Room Technique,* Phillips, N., 10th ed., 2004, page 520.

15. Documentation of ethylene oxide (EO) sterilizer cycle performance should describe the essential parameters for sterilization that include temperature, exposure time, humidity, and:
A. item being sterilized.
B. type of aerator.
C. sterilant concentration.
D. packaging being used.

Reference: *Standards, Recommended Practices and Guidelines,* AORN, Inc., 2006, page 633.

16. A patient receives midazolam (Versed), 2 mg IV during local anesthesia. Which of the following patient responses should the perioperative nurse expect to observe?
A. deviation in heart rate and respiratory depression.
B. increase in blood pressure and dizziness.
C. tachycardia and seizure activity.
D. hypotension, mild amnesia, and sedation.

Reference: *Moderate Sedation Competency Assessment Module,* CCI, 2005, page 21.

17. Flash sterilization should be considered only:
A. if the instruments are placed in an open tray with a wire mesh bottom and covered with a towel.
B. when there is insufficient time to process by the preferred wrapped or container method.
C. for instruments or materials made of metal.
D. for the sterilization of non-disposable items.

Reference: *Standards, Recommended Practices and Guidelines,* AORN, Inc., 2006, page 631.

18. When doing the preoperative skin preparation on an abdominal case, the perioperative nurse should start at the:
A. nipples and proceed toward the pubis.
B. site of incision to the periphery.
C. incision site and proceed upwards to nipples.
D. umbilicus and proceed in circles around it.

Reference: *Berry and Kohn's Operating Room Technique,* Phillips, N., 10th ed., 2004, page 496.

19. Proper surgical attire for non-scrubbed personnel includes:
A. home laundered scrub suit.
B. a double surgical mask.
C. sterile single-use gloves.
D. a long-sleeved jacket closed in front.

Reference: *Standards, Recommended Practices and Guidelines,* AORN, Inc., 2006, page 452.

20. All of the following statements are true regarding a patient with a do-not-resuscitate (DNR) order except?
A. If DNR orders are suspended intraoperatively, documentation should include when then the DNR order is to be reinstated.
B. The patient may completely or partially suspend their DNR orders during surgery.
C. A perioperative nurse with moral objections may find a substitute for the procedure.
D. DNR orders are automatically suspended upon entrance to the operating room.

Reference: *Standards, Recommended Practices and Guidelines,* AORN, Inc., 2006, pages 353-354.

21. Smoke evacuation systems used for plume generated during electrosurgery or laser use include all of the following except:
A. in-line.
B. individual evacuator.
C. centralized system.
D. high-flow insufflator.

Reference: *Alexander's Care of the Patient in Surgery,* Rothrock, J.C., 12th ed, 2003, pages 82-83.

22. All of the following are desirable characteristics of an antimicrobial agent for surgical scrubbing except:
A. fast acting.
B. broad-spectrum.
C. non-irritating to the skin.
D. reduction of all microorganisms.

Reference: *Standards, Recommended Practices and Guidelines,* AORN, Inc., 2006, page 539.

23. A perioperative nurse is circulating during a total joint replacement. It is most important for the nurse to document:
A. the lot number, manufacturer, and type of prosthesis.
B. that the legs were placed in adduction and externally rotated.
C. the manufacturer and sterilization method of the prosthesis.
D. the prep solution, site, and length of prep.

Reference: *Standards, Recommended Practices and Guidelines,* AORN, Inc., 2006, page 30.

24. At the start of the closure on a left lower lobectomy, the perioperative nurse and scrub nurse complete the first count and discover that a sponge is missing. The nurse's first action would be to:
A. repeat the count.
B. contact radiology.
C. document the incident.
D. notify the supervisor.

Reference: *Berry and Kohn's Operating Room Technique,* Phillips, N., 10th ed., 2004, page 462.

25. The provision of appropriate supplies and equipment needed to perform a procedure is an example of:
A. outcome identification.
B. implementation.
C. planning.
D. evaluation.

Reference: *Standards, Recommended Practices and Guidelines,* AORN, Inc., 2006, page 399.

Appendix II

Answer Key to Practice Questions

1.	A
2.	C
3.	A
4.	D
5.	B
6.	B
7.	A
8.	B
9.	C
10.	B
11.	B
12.	D
13.	B
14.	A
15.	C
16.	D
17.	B
18.	B
19.	D
20.	D
21.	D
22.	D
23.	A
24.	A
25.	C

Appendix III

Glossary of Terms

Accountable
The state of being answerable to self, patient, profession, and agency for nursing care given in the operating room.

Advanced Directive
A patient's signed and witnessed directive regarding health care, life-sustaining, and end-of-life decisions.

Ambulatory Surgery
For purposes of this document, outpatient surgery, same-day surgery, day surgery, etc, are included in the term "ambulatory surgery."

American Nurses Association (ANA)
ANA is the professional organization representing registered nurses. The ANA promulgates the *Code of Ethics with Interpretive Statements (see below)* that articulates the moral commitment to maintain the values and ethical obligations of all nurses. (www.ana.org).

AORN Standards, Recommended Practices, and Guidelines
As used in the Job Analysis, this term includes all sections of the *Standards, Recommended Practices, and Guidelines* published annually by AORN. The most current edition should be used at all times.

Assessment
Collecting data about a patient to determine the appropriate nursing diagnosis and expected outcomes. Includes patient's history and physical, vital signs, and all aspects of presenting condition. Assessment begins with data collection and ends with the formation of nursing diagnoses. Assessment is ongoing during the perioperative period (i.e., includes preoperative, intraoperative, postoperative).

Association for the Advancement of Medical Instrumentation (AAMI)
An organization with the goal of increasing the understanding and beneficial use of medical instrumentation. AAMI is the primary source of consensus and timely information on medical instrumentation and technology and is the primary resource for the industry, the professions, and government for national and international standards. (www.aami.org)

Association of periOperative Registered Nurses (AORN)
AORN is the professional organization of perioperative registered nurses that supports registered nurses in achieving optimal outcomes for patients undergoing operative and other invasive procedures. (www.aorn.org)

Autonomy
In the context of health care, autonomy is the patient's self-determination or ability and power to make his or her own decisions regarding health care.

Centers for Disease Control and Prevention (CDC)
The federal government agency dedicated to monitoring disease and mortality and morbidity of patients in the United States. This agency sets guidelines on dealing with known or suspected diseases. The CDC serves as the national focus for developing and applying disease prevention and control, environmental health, and health promotion and education activities designed to improve the health of the people of the United States. (www.cdc.gov)

Certification
The documented validation of the professional achievement of identified standards of practice of an individual registered nurse providing patient care before, during, and after surgery.

Code of Ethics
Guidelines regarding professional behavior and ethical decision making developed by the ANA. AORN has developed "explications for perioperative nursing" for each statement in the ANA code to provide the context within which perioperative nurses can make ethical decisions.

Community Resources
Other agencies that the perioperative nurse may refer patients to for special needs (e.g., American Cancer Society, American Heart Association, home health care agencies, social services, organ procurement agencies).

Competency
The knowledge, skills, and abilities necessary to fulfill assigned job functions.

Continuous Quality Assessment and Improvement
The continuous monitoring and evaluation of activities and services to improve the delivery of health care.

Continuum of Care
Care of patients undergoing operative or other invasive procedures is planned and implemented along a continuum—from the time the decision to undergo surgery is made, through the intraoperative period, and for an undetermined postoperative period until the patient's health status is improved or a specified health goal is reached.

Cultural Diversity
Perioperative nurses must be aware of the variety of backgrounds, beliefs, values, and ethnicity among patients. This diversity plays a major role in the communication efforts and actions of perioperative nurses. Every patient must be evaluated for individual cultural considerations in the perioperative setting.

Delegation
The transfer of responsibility for the performance of an activity from one individual to another while retaining accountability for the outcome.

Demonstration/Return Demonstration
The act of teaching that involves the visible, active demonstration of an activity, then involving the learner by having them demonstrate the identical activity back to the teacher.

Discharge Planning
The process of assessing the needs of patients for post-procedure care; developing a coordinated and multidisciplinary plan to provide the care required (including patient/family education, available services, and referral agencies and/or support groups); and evaluating the plan. The process begins before or on admission to the health care facility.

Documentation
The written record of nursing care including patient assessment, the actions taken as a result of that assessment, the plan of care developed and implemented, and the results of those actions. Documentation serves as the main, retrievable communication tool for the health care team.

Domain (related to certification)
A categorization of job responsibilities that includes the functions and tasks performed by perioperative nurses. Used for designing the certification examination.

Domain (related to the PNDS)
The four overall divisions of the conceptual framework of the *Perioperative Nursing Data Set*. All interventions and expected outcomes relate to one or more domain. The four domains are "Safety," "Physiologic Responses," "Behavioral Responses," and the "Health System."

Ergonomics
An applied science concerned with designing and arranging things (e.g., furniture, equipment) so that people can use the items efficiently and safely.

Extraneous Objects
Considered to be all equipment and supplies in the operating room, other than the patient and the health care team members. Includes all devices used, attached to the patient, or available in the room.

Family
For purposes of this document, the terms significant others and extended family are included in the term "family."

First Assistant (RN)
The RN first assistant (RNFA) at surgery collaborates with the surgeon and the health care team in performing a safe operation with optimal outcomes for the patient. The RNFA practices perioperative nursing and must have acquired the necessary knowledge, skills, and judgment specific to clinical practice. The RNFA practices in collaboration with and at the direction of the surgeon during the intraoperative phase of the perioperative experience. The RNFA does not concurrently function as a scrub nurse. *(AORN's "Official Statement on RN First Assistants.")*

Health Care Team
The providers of patient care services who are required to provide direct patient care to help the patient achieve a positive outcome. Support services include, but are not limited to, pharmacy, radiology, blood bank, housekeeping, etc.

Healthcare Insurance Portability and Accountability Act (HIPAA)
Legislation passed in 1996 that addresses various aspects of the use of patients' medical information, including confidentiality of patient information in the medical record, consent processes for access to patients' health information, and the right to sue the health plan provider.

Hyperthermia
See Malignant Hyperthermia

Hypothermia
A body temperature significantly below normal (i.e., 98.6° F [37° C]). May be caused by the operating room environment (e.g., room temperature, exposed skin) and can interfere with patient's maintenance of a normal physiologic state.

Informed Consent
The patient's right to make his or her own informed decisions based on information regarding treatment options, including the benefits, expected outcomes, and risk and potential complications; right to refuse treatment; and decisions regarding participation in research studies.

Intervention (Nursing)
Action taken, based on patient assessment data, with the intention of achieving one or more expected patient outcome.

Intraoperative Phase
Begins when the patient is transferred to the operating room bed and ends when he or she is admitted to the postanesthesia care unit.

Jehovah's Witness
A religious order whose members do not believe in the value or accept the transfusion of blood or blood products.

Job Analysis
The CCI Job Analysis describes the overall functions and responsibilities as well as the underlying knowledge and skills that are essential to ensure proficiency as a perioperative nurse.

Joint Commission on Accreditation of Healthcare Organizations (JCAHO)
The independent accrediting organization that designates acceptable patient care and evaluates health care facilities' abilities to adhere to specific guidelines (e.g., documentation, processes, policies, procedures). (www.jointcommission.org)

Knowledge
Defined as an organized body of information, usually of a factual or procedural nature, which, if applied, makes adequate performance of a job possible. Possession of knowledge does not ensure its proper application.

Malignant Hyperthermia
The rapid onset of extremely high fever with muscle rigidity, precipitated by exogenous agents in genetically susceptible people. Malignant hyperthermia is a complication of general anesthesia that occurs often without preexisting symptoms or warning.

Minimally Invasive Surgery
Surgery not requiring traditional incisions (i.e., performed through ports through which instrumentation are introduced).

Nonmaleficence
In the context of health care, acting in the best interest of the patient for the benefit of the patient.

North American Nursing Diagnosis Association (NANDA)
The group that has developed a list of 155 accepted nursing diagnoses to ensure that documentation in all areas of nursing use consistent, comparable terminology. (www.nanda.org)
Also see Perioperative Nursing Data Set.

Nursing Diagnosis
A statement derived from the nursing assessment data that provides the framework for nursing interventions that enable the patient to attain specific desired outcomes. It is structured using standardized nursing nomenclature.
Also see NANDA and Perioperative Nursing Data Set.

Nursing Process
The critical thinking a nurse uses to assess the health status of patients, identify problems, develop and implement plans of care, and evaluate the patients' responses to that care.

Occupational Safety and Health Administration (OSHA)
The federal government agency (a division of the US Department of Labor) that sets standards for and investigates the proper physical condition of working environments. OSHA's mission is to ensure safe and healthful workplaces in the United States. (www.osha.gov)

Outcome Criteria
Statements developed to identify the tasks or conditions to be implemented that will assist the patient in achieving the desired outcomes. Outcome criteria indicate an expected, measurable change in the patient's health status.

Patients' Rights
Every patient has the right to seek and receive health care regardless of his or her race, religion, or culture

and with respect for the individual's self-image, privacy, and other such considerations, in accordance with the Patients' Bill of Rights.

Perioperative Nursing Data Set (PNDS)
The structured and standardized vocabulary of perioperative nursing care, including perioperative nursing diagnoses, interventions, and outcome statements. This vocabulary, developed by AORN, has been recognized by the ANA as useful in clinical practice.

Perioperative Period
Time commencing with the decision for surgical intervention and ending with a follow-up home/clinic evaluation. This period includes the preoperative, intraoperative, and postoperative phases.

Plan of Care (or Care Plan)
A result of a systematic process of identifying expected patient outcomes and determining how to achieve them. It includes the list of interventions necessary to reach the expected outcome. The plan of care directs all nursing care activities related to each patient.

Postoperative Phase
Begins with admission to the postanesthesia care area and ends with the resolution of surgical sequelae.

Preoperative Phase
Begins when the decision for surgical intervention is made and ends with the transfer of the patient to the operating room bed.

Professional Achievement
The attainment of a measurable level of performance. In the context of CNOR certification, the level is set on a continuum between competency and excellence in perioperative nursing. Professional achievement affirms that the perioperative nurse demonstrates consistent application of the nursing process and the identified specialty standards of practice.

Regulatory Standards
CDC and OSHA regulations and standards and federal, state, and local laws/regulations that govern practice.

Safe Environment
The setting in which the physical and psychological aspects of the environment are controlled for the purpose of presenting the least possible hazard to the patient, staff members, and community.

Sentinel Event
An unexpected occurrence involving death or serious physical or psychological injury, or the risk thereof.

Significant Other
See Family

Skill
Defined as the proficient manual, verbal, or mental manipulation of data, people, or things. Skill embodies observable, quantifiable, and measurable performance parameters.

Standard Precautions
As used in the Job Analysis, this term refers to the standard and transmission-based precautions policies and procedures as developed by the CDC and OSHA.

Supervision
The active process of directing, guiding, and influencing the outcome of an individual's performance of an activity.

Support Services
Pharmacy, radiology, blood bank, laboratories, environmental services (i.e., housekeeping), biomedical engineering, etc.

Surgical Intervention
The patient's experiences during the preoperative, intraoperative, and postoperative phases including the technical aspects and anatomical approach.

Surgical Procedure
The technical aspects and anatomical approach used during surgical intervention.

Teaching/Learning Theories and Techniques
Those aids and methods that facilitate learning (e.g., audiovisual tools, return demonstration, adult learning principles).

"Time Out"
As an integral component of JCAHO's Universal Protocol for Preventing Wrong Site, Wrong Procedure, Wrong Person Surgery, a "time out" surgical site verification must be conducted in the location where the procedure will be done, just before starting the procedure. It must involve the entire operative team, use active communication, be briefly documented and must include, at the least:

- Correct patient identity
- Correct side and site
- Agreement on the procedure to be done
- Correct patient position
- Availability of correct implants and any special equipment or requirements

Processes and systems should be in place for reconciling differences in staff responses during the "time out."

Transfer

Moving a patient from one place to another (e.g., to or from a bed or stretcher, the stretcher to OR bed).

Transport

Moving a patient via a device (e.g., wheelchair, stretcher, wagon).

Unlicensed Assistive Personnel

Individuals who are trained to function in an assistive role to the registered nurse in providing patient care activities as delegated by, and under the supervision of, the registered nurse.

Voluntary Guidelines and Standards

AORN and JCAHO standards and recommended practices designed to provide guidelines for optimal levels of practice.

Appendix IV

Bibliography/References

The following references are cited in the text and are listed in alphabetical order.

Agency for Healthcare Research and Quality (AHRQ). *Glossary*. Available at: http://psnet.ahrq.gov/glossary.aspx. Accessed May 27. 2006.

Agency for Healthcare Research and Quality (AHRQ). *Training of Hospital Staff to Respond to a Mass Casualty Incident*. AHRQ PB04-E015-2. Rockville, MD: AHRQ; 2004.

American Hospital Association. *A Patient's Bill of Rights*. Available at: http://www.patienttalk.info/AHA-Patient_Bill_of_Rights.htm. Accessed September 19, 2006.

American Institute of Architects. *Guidelines for design and construction of hospital and health care facilities*. Washington, DC: The American Institute of Architects; 2001.

American National Standards Institute. ANSI Z136.3 *Safe Use of Lasers in Health Care Facilities*. Orlando, FL: Laser Institute of America; 1996.

American Nurses Association (ANA). *Code of Ethics for Nurses with Interpretive Statements*. Silver Spring, MD: American Nurses Association; 2001.

American Nurses Association (ANA). *Nursing Scope & Standards of Practice*. Silver Spring, MD: American Nurses Association; 2004.

American Nurses Association (ANA). *Nursing's Social Policy Statement*. Silver Spring, MD: American Nurses Association; 2003.

American Nurses Credentialing Center (ANCC). *The Magnet Recognition Program: Application Manual - 2005*. Silver Spring, MD: American Nurses Credentialing Center; 2005.

American Speech-Language-Hearing Assocation (ASHA), "Hospital noise stresses patients and staff." *The ASHA Leader*. 2006; 11(3): 5.

Arrowsmith VA, Maunder JA, Sargent RJ, Taylor R. "Removal of nail polish and ringer rings to prevent surgical infection." *Cochrane Database Syst Rev.* 2001;(4): CD003325.

Association for the Advancement of Medical Instrumentation (AAMI). *About AAMI*. Available at: http://www.aami.org/about/index.html. Accessed August 18, 2006.

Association of periOperative Registered Nurses (AORN). AORN *Standards, Recommended Practices, and Guidelines*. Denver, CO: AORN, Inc; 2006.

Association of periOperative Registered Nurses (AORN). AORN Online: *Workplace Safety: Ergonomics*. Available at: http://www.aorn.org/workplace/ergo.asp. Accessed August 10, 2006.

Beyea S, ed. *Perioperative Nursing Data Set: The Perioperative Nursing Vocabulary,* 2nd ed. Denver, CO: AORN, Inc; 2002.

Centers for Disease Control and Prevention (CDC). *About CDC: Mission*. Available at: http://www.cdc.gov/about/mission.htm. Accessed August 29, 2006.

Centers for Disease Control and Prevention (CDC). "Guideline for hand hygiene in healthcare settings; Recommendations of the Healthcare Infection Control Practices Advisory Committee and the HICPAC/SHEA/APIC/IDSA Hand Hygiene Task Force." Available at: http://www.cdc.gov/mmwr/preview/mmwrhtml/rr5116a1.htm. Accessed August 17, 2006.

Centers for Disease Control and Prevention (CDC). "Guideline for prevention of surgical site infection, 1999." Available at: http://www.cdc.gov/ncidod/dhqp/gl_surgicalsite.html. Accessed August 17, 2006.

Centers for Disease Control and Prevention (CDC). "Guidelines for prevention of surgical wound infections, 1985." Available at: http://www.cdc.gov/wonder/prevguid/p0000420/p0000420. Accessed September 15th, 2006.

Centers for Medicare and Medicaid Services (CMS). *Hospital quality initiatives*. Available at: http://www.cms.hhs.gov/HospitalQualityInits/01_Overview.asp. Accessed July 6, 2006.

Delbanco S. Commentary: "Improving quality and safety of healthcare delivery from the payer's perspective." Available at: http://www.unitedhealthfoundation.org/download/leapfrog.pdf. Accessed May 23, 2006.

Devaney l, Rowell KS. "Improving surgical wound classification—Why it matters." *AORN J.* 2004; 80(2): 208-223.

Doenges ME, Moorhouse MF, Geissler-Murr AC. *Nurse's Pocket Guide: Diagnoses, Interventions, and Rationales,* 9th ed. Philadelphia, PA: F. A. Davis; 2004.

ECRI. "A clinician's guide to surgical fires: How they occur, how to prevent them, how to put them out." *Health Devices* 2003; 32(1): 5-24. Available at: http://www.guideline.gov/summary/summary.aspx?doc_id=3688&nbr=2914. Accessed August 18, 2006.

ECRI. *About ECRI, our mission*. Available at: http://www.ecri.org/About_ECRI/About_ECRI.aspx#Mission. Accessed August 17, 2006.

Eiland JE, Pritchard DA, Stevens DA. "Emergency preparedness—is your OR ready?" *AORN J.* 2004;79(6):1276-83.

Fogg, DM. "Infection prevention and control." In *Alexander's Care of the Patient in Surgery*, 12th ed. J. Rothrock, ed. St. Louis, MO: Mosby, Inc; 2003; 97-158.

Gabel RA, Kulli JC, Lee BS, Spratt DG, Ward DS. *Operating Room Management.* Woburn, MA: Butterworth-Heinemann; 1999.

Georgia Nurses Association. *Nurse Advocate Program.* Available at: http://www.georgianurses.org/impaired_nurse.htm. Accessed August 11, 2006.

Griffitts LD. "Geared to achieve with lifelong learning." *Nurs Manage*. 2002;33(11):22-5.

Gronert GA, Pessah IN, Muldoon SM, Tautz TJ. "Malignant hyperthermia." In *Miller's Anesthesia*, 6th ed. RD Miller, ed. Philadelphia, PA: Elsevier; 2005; 1169-1190.

Gruendemann BJ, Mangum SS. *Infection Prevention in Surgical Settings*. Philadelphia, PA: WB Saunders Co; 2001; 282-284.

Health care quality: *Patient Rights and Responsibilities.* Available at: http://www.consumer.gov/qualityhealth/rights.htm. Accessed May 25, 2006.

Healthcare Infection Control Practices Advisory Committee (HICPAC). *About HICPAC*. Available at: http://www.cdc.gov/ncidod/dhqp/hicpac.html. Accessed August 29, 2006.

Ignatavicius DD, Workman ML. *Medical-Surgical Nursing: Critical Thinking for Collaborative Care*, 5th ed. St. Louis: Elsevier Saunders; 2006.

Institute for Healthcare Improvement (IHI). *Patient-Centered Care.* Available at: http://www.ihi.org/IHI/Topics/PatientCenteredCare. Accessed July 31, 2006.

Institute for Healthcare Improvement (IHI). *SBAR Technique for Communication: A Situational Briefing Model*. Available at: http://www.ihi.org/IHI/Topics/PatientSafety/SafetyGeneral/Tools/SBARTechniqueforCommunicationASituationalBriefingModel.htm. Accessed October 19, 2006.

Institutes of Medicine. *To Err is Human: Building a Safer Health System*. November 1999. Available at: http://www.iom.edu/Object.File/Master/4/117/ToErr-8pager.pdf. Accessed July 24, 2006.

Joint Commission on Accreditation of Healthcare Organizations (JCAHO). *Comprehensive Manual for Hospitals,* Oakbrook Terrace, IL: JCAHO; 2006.

Joint Commission on Accreditation of Healthcare Organizations (JCAHO). *Facts About the Joint Commission on Accreditation of Healthcare Organizations.* Available at: http://www.jointcommission.org/AboutUs/joint_commission_facts.htm. Accessed: August 19, 2006.

Joint Commission on Accreditation of Healthcare Organizations (JCAHO). *2006 Hospital Accreditation Standards for Emergency Management Planning, Emergency Management Drills, Infection Control, Disaster Privileges.* Available at: http://www.jointcommission.org/NR/rdonlyres/F42AF828-7248-48C0-B4E6-BA18E719A87C/0/06_hap_accred_stnds.pdf. Accessed June 2, 2006.

Joint Commission on Accreditation of Healthcare Organizations (JCAHO). *2007 Hospital/Critical Access Hospital National Patient Safety Goals.* Available at: http://www.jointcommission.org/PatientSafety/NationalPatientSafetyGoals/07_hap_cah_npsgs.htm. Accessed November 22, 2006.

Joint Commission on Accreditation of Healthcare Organizations (JCAHO). *Introduction to the National*

Patient Safety Goals. Available at: http://www.joint commmission.org/PatientSafety/NationalPatientSafetyGoals/npsg_intro.htm. Accessed June 8, 2006.

Joint Commission on Accreditation of Healthcare Organizations (JCAHO). *Patient Safety and Universal Protocol.* Available at: http://www.jointcommission.org/PatientSafety/UniversalProtocol/up_faqs.htm. Accessed September 18, 2006.

Joint Commission on Accreditation of Healthcare Organizations (JCAHO. *The Joint Commission Guide to Improving Staff Communication.* Oakbrook Terrace, IL: Joint Commission Resources; 2005.

Joint Commission on Accreditation of Healthcare Organizations (JCAHO). *Universal Protocol for Preventing Wrong Site, Wrong Procedure, Wrong Person Surgery.* Available at: http://www.jointcommission.org/NR/rdonlyres/E3C600EB-043B-4E86-B04E-CA4A89AD5433/0/universal_protocol.pdf. Accessed August 10, 2006.

Kleinbeck S. *PNDS @ Work.* Denver, CO: AORN, Inc; 2005.

Kleinbeck SV, Dopp A. "The perioperative nursing data set—A new language for documenting care." *AORN J.* 2005; 82(1):51-57.

Kristeller AR. "Medical staff: privileging and credentialing." *New Jersey Medicine.* 1995; 92 (1): 26 -28.

Leiper J. "Nurse against nurse: how to stop horizontal violence." *Nursing.* 2005;35(3):44-5.

Lemone P, Burke K. *Medical-Surgical Nursing: Critical Thinking in Client Care*, 3rd ed. Upper Saddle River, NJ: Pearson Prentice Hall; 2004.

Linck C, Phillips S. "Managing disruptive behavior on an acute medical/surgical service: A strategy for success." *Holistic Nursing Practice.* 2004; 18(5): 223-27.

Luby M, Riley JK, Towne G. "Nursing research journal clubs: bridging the gap between practice and research." *Medsurg Nurs.* 2006;15(2):100-2.

Maguire T. "Barriers to communication—how things go wrong." *The Pharmaceutical Journal.* February 23, 2002; 268. Available at: http://www.pjonline.com/pdf/cpd/pj_20020223_communication1.pdf. Accessed June 1, 2006.

Maguire T. "Good communication—how to get it right." *The Pharmaceutical Journal.* March 2, 2002; 268. Available at: http://www.pjonline.com/pdf/cpd/pj_20020302_commun ication2.pdf. Accessed June 1, 2006.

Malignant Hyperthermia Association of the United States. http://www.mhaus.org. Accessed May 30, 2006.

Mangram AJ, Horan TC, Pearson ML, Silver LC, Jarvis WR. "Guideline for prevention of surgical site infection, 1999." *Infect Control Hosp Epidemiol.* 1999; 20(4):250-78.

Mazer SE. "Hear, hear. Assessing and resolving hospital noise issues." *Health Facil Manage.* 2005;18(4):24-9.

McGlinch BP, White RD. "Cardiopulmonary resuscitation: Basic and advanced life support." In *Miller's Anesthesia,* 6th ed. RD Miller, ed. Philadelphia, PA: Elsevier; 2005; 2923-2954.

MedQIC (Medicare Quality Improvement Community). Available at: http://www.medqic.org/dcs/ContentServer?cid=1089815967030&pagename=Medqic%2FContent%2FParentShellTemplate&parentName=Topic&c=MQParents. Accessed August 17, 2006.

Moolenaar RL, Crutcher JM, San Joaquin VH, Sewell LV, Hutwagner LC, Carson LA, Robison DA, Smithee LM, Jarvis WR. "A prolonged outbreak of Pseudomonas aeruginosa in a neonatal intensive care unit: Did staff fingernails play a role in disease transmission?" *Infect Control Hosp* Epidemiol. 2000;21(2):80-5.

Moore, DT. "National Patient Safety Goals; do-not-use abbreviations; tissue banking; patient skin preparation; patient attire." (Clinical Issues) *AORN J.* 2005. Available at: http://www.aorn.org/journal/2005/augci.htm#2. Accessed September 18, 2006.

Moorhead S, Johnson M, Maas, M. *Nursing Outcomes Classification (NOC)*, 3rd ed. St. Louis: Mosby; 2004.

Murphy J. "Temperature & humidity control in surgery rooms." *RX for Health-Care HVAC - A Supplement to ASHRAE Journal.* 2006; 48: H18-24.

National Institute for Occupational Safety and Health (NIOSH). *About NIOSH.* Available at: http://www.cdc.gov/niosh/about.html. Accessed August 19, 2006.

National Patient Safety Foundation. *Agenda for research and development in patient safety.* Chicago, IL: NPSF; 2000.

National Patient Safety Foundation. *Roundtable discussion: Reporting as a means to improve patient safety.* March 16-17, 2000. Available at: http://www.npsf.org/download/patientsafetyroundtable.pdf. Accessed May 27, 2006.

North American Nursing Diagnosis Association (NANDA). NANDA-I. Available at: http://www.nanda.org/html/about.html. Accessed October 18, 2006.

Owen BD. "Preventing injuries using an ergonomic approach." *AORN J.* 2000;72(6):1030-1036.

Peterson C. *Leadership in Action: A Manager's Guide to Success.* Denver, CO: AORN, Inc.: 2004.

Phillips NF. *Berry & Kohn's Operating Room Technique,* 10th ed. NF Phillips, ed. St Louis, MO: Mosby; 2004.

Pizzi L, Goldfarb N, Nash D. "Promoting a culture of safety." In Shojania KG, Duncan BW, McDonald KM, Wachter RM, eds. *Making Health Care Safer: A Critical Analysis of Patient Safety Practices.* Evidence Report/ Technology Assessment No. 43 from the Agency for Healthcare Research and Quality: AHRQ Publication No. 01-E058; 2001. Available at: http://www.ncbi.nlm.nih.gov/books/bv.fcgi?rid=hstat1.section.61719. Accessed May 27, 2006.

Polit DF, Beck CT, Hungler BP. *Essentials of Nursing Research: Methods, Appraisal, and Utilization,* 5th ed. Philadelphia, PA: Lippincott; 2001.

Porth, CM. *Pathophysiology: Concepts of Altered Health States,* 5th ed. CM. Porth. Philadelphia: PA; Lippincott; 1998; 335-362.

Rothrock J. *Perioperative Nursing Care Planning,* 2nd edition. St. Louis, MO: CV Mosby Company; 1996.

Rothrock JC. *Alexander's Care of the Patient in Surgery,* 12th ed. J. Rothrock, ed. St. Louis, MO: Mosby, Inc; 2003.

Rothrock, JC, Smith, DA. "Patient and Environmental Safety." In *Alexander's Care of the Patient in Surgery,* 12th ed. J Rothrock, ed. St Louis, MO: Mosby, Inc; 2003; 17-40.

Silva MC, Ludwick, R. "Is the doctor of nursing practice ethical?" *Online J Issues Nurs.* 2006; 11(2). Available at: http://www.medscape.com/nurses/journals?cid=med. Accessed August 11, 2006.

Simunek LCA. "Legal and ethical dimensions of perioperative nursing practice." In *Perioperative Nursing: Principles and Practice,* 2nd ed. S.S. Fairchild, ed. Philadelphia, PA: Little, Brown and Company (Inc.); 1996; 378-404.

Spry, C. *Essentials of Perioperative Nursing,* 3rd ed. C Spry, ed . Sudbury, MA; Jones and Bartlett Publishers; 2005; 1-7.

Stauder T. *Sharpening your management skills.* Available at: http://www.stsc.hill.af.mil/crosstalk/1999/07/publisher.asp. Accessed August 10, 2006.

Sword SLH. "The surgical setting - Unit 2 - Organizational structure: The team concept." In *Perioperative Nursing: Principles and Practice,* 2nd ed. S.S. Fairchild, ed. Philadelphia, PA: Little, Brown and Company (Inc.); 1996; 24-32.

Trick WE, Vernon MO, Hayes RA, Nathan C, Rice TW, Peterson BJ, Segreti J, Welbel SF, Solomon SL, Weinstein RA. "Impact of ring wearing on hand contamination and comparison of hand hygiene agents in a hospital." *Clin Infect Dis.* 2003;36(11):1383-90.

US Department of Justice, Drug Enforcement Administration, Office of Diversion Control. *Drug Addition in Health Care Professionals.* Available at: http://www.deadiversion.usdoj.gov/pubs/brochures/drug_hc.htm. Accessed June 2, 2006.

US Department of Labor, Occupational Health and Safety Administration (OSHA). Available at http://www.osha.gov. Accessed May 23, 2006.

U.S. Department of Labor, Occupational Safety and Health Administration (OSHA). *Ergonomics.* Available at: http://www.osha.gov/SLTC/etools/hospital/hazards/ergo/ergo.html. Accessed June 19, 2006.

US Department of Labor, Occupational Safety and Health Administration (OSHA). Hazard communication: 1910.1200. *Toxic and hazardous substances.* Available at: http://www.osha.gov/pls/oshaweb/owadisp.show_document?p_table=STANDARDS&p_id=10099. Accessed June 1, 2006.

United States Department of Labor, Occupational Safety and Health Administration (OSHA). *OSHA's mission.* Available at: http://www.osha.gov/oshinfo/mission.html. Accessed August 19, 2006.

United States Department of Veteran Affairs. *Operating room air distribution.* Available at: http://www.va.gov/facmgt/consulting/orair.asp. Accessed August 5, 2006.

United States Food and Drug Administration. *Tissue Action Plan.* Available at: http://www.fda.gov/cber/tissue/tissue.htm.

VanCura BJ, Gunchick D. "Five key components for effectively working with unlicensed assistive personnel." *Medsurg Nurs.* 1997;6(5):270-4.

Appendix V
Recommended Study Material

In addition to the references cited in the bibliography, the following is a list of recommended study material that may also be useful in preparing for the exam.

AAMI. *AAMI Standards and Recommended Practices - Volume 1: Sterilization.* Arlington, VA: Association for the Advancement of Medical Instrumentation; 2003.

AAMI. *AAMI Standards and Recommended Practices - Volume 2: Biomedical Equipment.* Arlington, VA: Association for the Advancement of Medical Instrumentation; 2003.

Allen G. "Maximizing nurses' advocacy role to improve patient outcomes." *AORN J.* 2000; 71(5):1038-1050.

Beyea SC. "Structural data elements: Standardized terms and definitions." *AORN J.* 2000; 71(3):541-549.

Collette CL. "Understanding patients' needs is the foundation of perioperative nursing." *AORN J.* 2000; 71(3):629-630.

Dochterman JM, Bulechek GM, eds. *Nursing Interventions Classification (NIC),* 4th ed. St. Louis, MO: Mosby; 2004.

Drake B. "Infection control in hospitals." *RX for Health-Care HVAC - A Supplement to ASHRAE Journal.* 2006; 48: H12-17.

Ferguson L. "External validity, generalizability, knowledge utilization." *J Nurs Scholarsh.* 2004; 36(1):16-22.

Hewitt-Taylor J. "Evidence-based practice." *Nurs Stand.* 2002; 17(14-15):47-55.

Keenan G, Stocker J, Barkauskas V, Treder M, Heath C. "Toward collecting a standardized nursing data set across the continuum: case of adult care nurse practitioner setting." *Outcomes Manag.* 2003; 7(3):113-120.

Kirchner BA, Stewart D. *Ambulatory Surgery Safety Policies and Procedures.* Denver, CO: AORN, Inc; 2005.

Kleinbeck S. *PNDS @ Work: Building a Perioperative Patient Record.* Denver, CO: AORN, Inc. 2004.

Kleinpell R, Gawlinski A. "Assessing outcomes in advanced practice nursing practice: The use of quality indicators and evidence-based practice." *AACN Clin Issues.* 2005; 16(1):43-57.

Kuehl NK, Parker N, eds. *Ethics in Perioperative Practice.* Denver, CO: AORN, Inc; 2004.

Lipp A. "The systematic review as evidence-based tool for the operating room." *AORN J.* 2005; 81(6):1279-1287.

Lunney M, Parker L, Fiore L, Cavendish R, Pulcini J. "Feasibility of studying the effects of using NANDA, NIC, and NOC on nurses' power and children's outcomes." *Comput Inform Nurs.* 2004; 22(6):316-325.

Moss R, Smart T. *Perioperative Pharmacology Reference Book.* Denver, CO: CCI; 2006.

Patterson K, Grenny J, McMillan R, Switzler, A. *Crucial Confrontations.* New York, NY: McGraw-Hill. 2005.

Rothrock JC, Smith DA. "Selecting the perioperative patient focused model." *AORN J.* 2000; 71(5):1030-1037.

"Safety Net: Lessons Learned From Close Calls in the OR." *AORN J.* 2006; 84 (Supplement 1).

US Department of Health and Human Services. Office of Civil Rights. *Medical privacy - national standards to protect the privacy of personal health information.* Available at: http://www.hhs.gov/ocr/hipaa/. Accessed October 17, 2006.

US Department of Health and Human Services. *Protecting the privacy of patients' health information.* Available at: http://www.hhs.gov/news/facts/privacy.html. Accessed September 17, 2006.

US Department of Health and Human Services. *The Patients Bill of Rights in Medicare and Medicaid.* Available at: http://www.hhs.gov/news/press/1999pres/990412.html. Accessed October 17, 2006.

Notes

Notes

Notes

Notes

Notes